COMMANDO 90
Training Programme

Max Glover

First published in Great Britain in 2021 by Amazon
This edition published in 2023
2
Copyright © Max Glover 2021

The right of Max Glover to be identified as the Author of the Work has been asserted by him in accordance with the Copyright, Designs and Patents Act 1988.
The views and opinions expressed in this book are those of the author alone.
All rights reserved.
No part of this publication may be reproduced, stored in a retrieval system, or transmitted, in any form or by any means without the prior written permission.

ISBN 9798372852631

Independently published

Disclaimer:

1. Max Glover strongly recommends that you consult with your physician before beginning any exercise program. You should be in good physical condition and be able to participate in the exercise. Max Glover is not a licensed medical care provider and has no expertise in diagnosing, examining, or treating medical conditions of any kind, or in determining the effect of any specific exercise on a medical condition.
2. You should understand that when participating in any exercise or exercise program, there is the possibility of physical injury. If you engage in this exercise or exercise program, you agree that you do so at your own risk, are voluntarily participating in these activities, assume all risk of injury to yourself.
3. The information provided is not intended to be a substitute for professional medical advice, diagnosis or treatment. Never disregard professional medical advice, or delay in seeking it.
4. You are encouraged to consult with your doctor with regard to the information contained within this book.
5. Each individual's health, fitness, and nutrition success depends on his or her background, dedication, desire, and motivation. As with any health-related program or service, your results may vary, and will be based on many variables, including but not limited to, your individual capacity, life experience, unique health and genetic profile, starting point, expertise, and level of commitment.

Contents

Welcome 7
Programme Schedule 8
Day 1 11
Day 2 12
Day 3 12
Day 4 13
Day 5 13
Day 6 13
Day 7 14
Day 8 14
Day 9 15
Day 10 15
Day 11 15
Day 12 16
Day 13 17
Day 14 17
Day 15 18
Day 16 18
Day 17 18
Day 18 19
Day 19 19
Day 20 20
Day 21 20
Day 22 20
Day 23 21
Day 24 21
Day 25 21
Day 26 23

Day 27 23

Day 28 24

Day 29 24

Day 30 24

Day 31 25

Day 32 25

Day 33 26

Day 34 26

Day 35 26

Day 36 27

Day 37 27

Day 38 27

Day 39 28

Day 40 28

Day 41 29

Day 42 & 43 29

Day 44 30

Day 45 31

Day 46 31

Day 47 31

Day 48 32

Day 49 32

Day 50 32

Day 51 33

Day 52 34

Day 53 34

Day 54 34

Day 55 35

Day 56 35

Day 57 36

Day 58 36
Day 59 36
Day 60 37
Day 61 37
Day 62 37
Day 63 38
Day 64 38
Day 65 39
Day 66 39
Day 67 39
Day 68 40
Day 69 40
Day 70 & 71 41
Day 72 41
Day 73 43
Day 74 43
Day 75 44
Day 76 44
Day 77 44
Day 78 44
Day 79 45
Day 80 45
Day 81 46
Day 82 46
Day 83 46
Day 84 46
Day 85 47
Day 86 47
Day 87 47
Day 88 & 89 48

Day 90 .... **48**

Exercise Guide **50**

Stretching Guide **62**

Author Profile **66**

Welcome

Welcome to the Commando90 Training programme. This is a tough yet progressive programme that is inspired by military fitness routines. Before you begin training, please make sure that you are fit and well and have your doctor's permission to take part in an intense exercise programme.

Please read the programme details carefully, and pay attention to the supporting information.

If you have any injuries or medical conditions that could be negatively affected by an exercise programme please do not begin this programme.

You are responsible for ensuring that you are exercising in a safe environment, and make sure you wear appropriate exercise attire throughout. Some exercise alternatives (progressions / regressions) are included in the Exercise Guide section.

To be Successful follow these rules...

Warm Up
All workouts must begin with a thorough warm up, follow this procedure:
Raise blood flow, muscle temperature, core temperature, and muscle elasticity through low intensity movements
Activate & Mobilise Your muscles and joints with dynamic movements
Potentiate The movements you are doing in the workout, eg gradually increase the weight you are doing on a squat, or build up speed on short sprints

Hydration
It is imperative that you stay hydrated throughout the day by drinking plenty of water. The easiest way to stay on top of this is to check the colour of your urine. Ideally it should be clear or a pale yellow. If it's dark yellow you need to drink more water. Make sure that you have drinking water with you during your runs, circuits and load carries.

Safety
You are responsible for your route selection, it is advisable to select a route that is adequately lit, with good firm flooring and does not involve you going out on the road. You should wear high visibility clothing and appropriate training attire at all times. When going on a run / loaded march you should make others aware that you are going out, what you are doing, where you are going and an estimated time of return.

Injuries / Feeling Unwell
Pushing through a workout when you're injured or unwell is not smart and injuries are not a badge of honour. If at any point you feel unwell or become injured during this training programme you must stop immediately, contact your doctor and not resume the programme until you have had permission from a medical professional.

If you do need to stop or take additional breaks from this programme that is fine, there are scheduled rests in the programme but everyone is different and some people take longer to recover than others. You can insert additional rests in as you see fit and just carry the programme on from there.

Thank you for taking part in this programme, I wish you the very best on your journey!

Programme Schedule

Day	Programme Schedule
1	Fitness Tests
2	Circuit
3	4 Km Run
4	Strength Circuit
5	REST
6	Run – Hill Repeats
7	Circuit
8	4.5 Km Run
9	Strength Circuit
10	REST
11	Run – Hill Repeats
12	Circuit
13	5 Km Run
14	Strength Circuit
15	REST
16	Run – Hill Repeats
17	Circuit
18	5.5 Km Run
19	Strength Circuit
20	REST
21	Run – Hill Repeats
22	Circuit
23	REST
24	REST
25	Fitness Test
26	6 Km Run
27	Strength Circuit
28	REST
29	Tempo Run

30	Circuit
31	5.5 Km Run
32	Intensity Circuit
33	REST
34	Loaded March
35	Circuit
36	6 Km Steady Run
37	REST
38	Tempo Run
39	Circuit
40	6.5 Km Steady Run
41	Intensity Circuit
42	REST
43	REST
44	Fitness Test
45	REST
46	7 Km Steady Run
47	Circuit
48	Loaded March
49	REST
50	7.5 Km Steady Run
51	Intensity Circuit
52	Loaded March
53	REST
54	7 Km Steady Run
55	Circuit
56	Run - Hill Repeats
57	REST
58	7.5 Km Steady Run
59	Intensity Circuit
60	Loaded March
61	REST
62	Tempo Run
63	Circuit
64	Hill Repeats
65	REST

	66	8 Km Steady Run
	67	Intensity Circuit
	68	Loaded March
	69	Circuit
	70	REST
	71	REST
	72	Fitness Test
	73	9 Km Steady Run
	74	Circuit 3
	75	REST
	76	Loaded March
	77	Tempo Run + Mini Circuit
	78	REST
	79	9.5 Km Steady Run
	80	Circuit 3
	81	REST
	82	Loaded March
	83	Tempo Run + Mini Circuit
	84	REST
	85	10 Km Steady Run
	86	Circuit 3
	87	Run – Hill Repeats
	88	REST
	89	REST
	90	Fitness Test

A note on testing and exercise selection. If you are unable to complete 1 rep of an exercise such as press ups or pull ups… attempt the test and score ZERO. During your exercises and circuits use the assisted version of the exercise that is shown in the exercise guide. There are three alternatives that can be used for pull ups – band assisted pull up, body row and body row with rope. You will gradually get stronger.

Active Recovery – Perform non strenuous activity such as walking or gentle swimming.

Day 1

Test
Aerobic Fitness Test. This is a 12 minute test to measure the efficiency of your circulatory and respiratory system in supplying oxygen to your muscles during physical activity.

Spend 15 minutes warming up and then run as far as you can for 12 minutes. You will need to be able to track the distance you are running. This test is ideally performed on a running track, however a treadmill can be used (1% gradient must be applied).

Test Results
Male

Age	Excellent	Above Average	Average	Below Average	Poor
17-19	>3000m	2700-3000m	2500-2699m	2300-2499m	<2300m
20-29	>2800m	2400-2800m	2200-2399m	1600-2199m	<1600m
30-39	>2700m	2300-2700m	1900-2299m	1500-1899m	<1500m
40-49	>2500m	2100-2500m	1700-2099m	1400-1699m	<1400m
>50	>2400m	2000-2400m	1600-1999m	1300-1599m	<1300m

Female

Age	Excellent	Above Average	Average	Below Average	Poor
17-19	>2300m	2100-2300m	1800-2099m	1700-1799m	<1700m
20-29	>2700m	2200-2700m	1800-2199m	1500-1799m	<1500m
30-39	>2500m	2000-2500m	1700-1999m	1400-1699m	<1400m
40-49	>2300m	1900-2300m	1500-1899m	1200-1499m	<1200m
>50	>2200m	1700-2200m	1400-1699m	1100-1399m	<1100m

Muscular Fitness Test *(set 2 minute timer for press ups)*

Exercise	Excellent	Above Average	Average	Below Average	Poor
Press Ups	>60	40-60	25-39	10 – 24	<10
Pull Ups	>16	11 – 16	7 – 10	3 – 6	<2
Plank	>4:00	3:01 – 4:00	2:01 – 3:00	1:00 – 2:00	<1:00

Test	Your Score	Date	Target for next test
Cooper Test			
Press Ups			
Pull Ups			
Planks			

Day 2

Circuit

Warm Up
Gentle jog 5 mins (on the spot or on the move)
Mobilisation of joints – shoulder circles etc
30 jumping jacks
30 high knees
30 heel flicks
30 seconds jog on spot
5 second sprint on spot
Lying side leg lift x 20 each leg
Glute bridge x 20

30 seconds work 30 seconds rest. Do as many repetitions of each exercise with good form in 30 seconds, take 30 seconds rest and then perform that exercise again before moving on to the next exercise (30 seconds rest).

Burpees 30s x 2
Press ups 30s x 2
Squats 30s x 2
Pull ups 30s x 2
Alternate split squats 30s x 2
Shoulder press 30s x 2
Body row 30s x 2
Plank 30s x 2

Take 1 minute rest and then repeat.

Stretch

Day 3

Run
Warm Up
Gentle jog 5 mins (on the spot or on the move)
Mobilisation of joints – shoulder circles etc
30 jumping jacks
30 high knees
30 heel flicks
30 seconds jog on spot
5 second sprint on spot
Lying side leg lift x 20 each leg
Glute bridge x 20

4Km run steady pace. If you cannot run the full distance complete in run/walk fashion. **Stretch.**

Day 4

Strength Circuit (Or if opting for bodyweight perform circuit as on day 2)
Warm Up

Gentle jog 5 mins (on the spot or on the move)
Mobilisation of joints – shoulder circles etc
30 jumping jacks
30 high knees
30 heel flicks
30 seconds jog on spot
5 second sprint on spot
Lying side leg lift x 20 each leg
Glute bridge x 20

Squats 2 x 15 Dead lifts 2 x 10 Pull ups 2 x 10 Dips 2 x 10 Renegade row 2 x 10 (each side) Plank 2 x 35 seconds	Pick a weight that allows you to perform the target number of reps with good form stopping before failure

Stretch

Day 5

Rest day – must go for a gentle walk (active recovery)

Day 6

Hill repeats

Warm Up
Gentle jog 5 mins (on the spot or on the move)
Mobilisation of joints – shoulder circles etc
30 jumping jacks
30 high knees
30 heel flicks
30 seconds jog on spot
5 second sprint on spot
Lying side leg lift x 20 each leg
Glute bridge x 20

Once warm, run up a short hill and then walk down this is 1 set. Perform 6 sets at 100% effort.

Cool down with gentle jog / walk for 5 minutes

Stretch

Day 7

Circuit

Warm Up
Gentle jog 5 mins (on the spot or on the move)
Mobilisation of joints – shoulder circles etc
30 jumping jacks
30 high knees
30 heel flicks
30 seconds jog on spot
5 second sprint on spot
Lying side leg lift x 20 each leg
Glute bridge x 20

30 seconds work 30 seconds rest. Do as many repetitions of each exercise with good form in 30 seconds, take 30 seconds rest and then perform that exercise again before moving on to the next exercise (30 seconds rest).

Burpees 30s x 2
Press ups 30s x 2
Squats 30s x 2
Pull ups 30s x 2
Alternate split squats 30s x 2
Shoulder press 30s x 2
Body row 30s x 2
Plank 30s x 2

Take 1 minute rest and then repeat.

Stretch

Day 8

Run

Warm Up
Gentle jog 5 mins (on the spot or on the move)
Mobilisation of joints – shoulder circles etc
30 jumping jacks
30 high knees
30 heel flicks
30 seconds jog on spot

5 second sprint on spot
Lying side leg lift x 20 each leg
Glute bridge x 20

4.5Km run steady pace. If you cannot run the full distance complete in run/walk fashion.

Stretch

Day 9

Strength Circuit

Warm Up

Gentle jog 5 mins (on the spot or on the move)
Mobilisation of joints – shoulder circles etc
30 jumping jacks
30 high knees
30 heel flicks
30 seconds jog on spot
5 second sprint on spot
Lying side leg lift x 20 each leg
Glute bridge x 20

Squats 2 x 15 Dead lifts 2 x 10 Pull ups 2 x 10 Dips 2 x 10 Renegade row 2 x 10 (each side) Plank 2 x 40 seconds	Pick a weight that allows you to perform the target number of reps with good form stopping before failure

Stretch

Day 10

Rest day – must go for a gentle walk

Day 11

Hill repeats

Warm Up
Gentle jog 5 mins (on the spot or on the move)
Mobilisation of joints – shoulder circles etc
30 jumping jacks

30 high knees
30 heel flicks
30 seconds jog on spot
5 second sprint on spot
Lying side leg lift x 20 each leg
Glute bridge x 20

Once warm, run up a short hill and then walk down this is 1 set. Perform 6 sets at 100% effort.

Cool down with gentle jog / walk for 5 minutes

Stretch

Day 12

Circuit

Warm Up
Gentle jog 5 mins (on the spot or on the move)
Mobilisation of joints – shoulder circles etc
30 jumping jacks
30 high knees
30 heel flicks
30 seconds jog on spot
5 second sprint on spot
Lying side leg lift x 20 each leg
Glute bridge x 20

30 seconds work 30 seconds rest. Do as many repetitions of each exercise with good form in 30 seconds, take 30 seconds rest and then perform that exercise again before moving on to the next exercise (30 seconds rest).

Burpees 30s x 2
Press ups 30s x 2
Squats 30s x 2
Pull ups 30s x 2
Alternate split squats 30s x 2
Shoulder press 30s x 2
Body row 30s x 2
Plank 30s x 2

Take 1 minute rest and then repeat.

Stretch

Day 13

Run

Warm Up
Gentle jog 5 mins (on the spot or on the move)
Mobilisation of joints – shoulder circles etc
30 jumping jacks
30 high knees
30 heel flicks
30 seconds jog on spot
5 second sprint on spot
Lying side leg lift x 20 each leg
Glute bridge x 20

5Km run steady pace. If you cannot run the full distance complete in run/walk fashion.

Stretch

Day 14

Strength Circuit

Warm Up
Gentle jog 5 mins (on the spot or on the move)
Mobilisation of joints – shoulder circles etc
30 jumping jacks
30 high knees
30 heel flicks
30 seconds jog on spot
5 second sprint on spot
Lying side leg lift x 20 each leg
Glute bridge x 20

Squats 2 x 15 Dead lifts 2 x 10 Pull ups 2 x 10 Dips 2 x 10 Renegade row 2 x 10 (each side) Plank 2 x 45 seconds	Pick a weight that allows you to perform the target number of reps with good form stopping before failure

Stretch

Day 15

Rest day – must go for a gentle walk

Day 16

Hill repeats

Warm Up
Gentle jog 5 mins (on the spot or on the move)
Mobilisation of joints – shoulder circles etc
30 jumping jacks
30 high knees
30 heel flicks
30 seconds jog on spot
5 second sprint on spot
Lying side leg lift x 20 each leg
Glute bridge x 20

Once warm, run up a short hill and then walk down this is 1 set. Perform 6 sets at 100% effort.

Cool down with gentle jog / walk for 5 minutes

Stretch

Day 17

Circuit

Warm Up
Gentle jog 5 mins (on the spot or on the move)
Mobilisation of joints – shoulder circles etc
30 jumping jacks
30 high knees
30 heel flicks
30 seconds jog on spot
5 second sprint on spot
Lying side leg lift x 20 each leg
Glute bridge x 20

30 seconds work 30 seconds rest. Do as many repetitions of each exercise with good form in 30 seconds, take 30 seconds rest and then perform that exercise again before moving on to the next exercise (30 seconds rest).

Burpees 30s x 2
Press ups 30s x 2

Squats 30s x 2
Pull ups 30s x 2
Alternate split squats 30s x 2
Shoulder press 30s x 2
Body row 30s x 2
Plank 30s x 2

Take 1 minute rest and then repeat.

Stretch

Day 18

Run

Warm Up
Gentle jog 5 mins (on the spot or on the move)
Mobilisation of joints – shoulder circles etc
30 jumping jacks
30 high knees
30 heel flicks
30 seconds jog on spot
5 second sprint on spot
Lying side leg lift x 20 each leg
Glute bridge x 20

5.5Km run steady pace. If you cannot run the full distance complete in run/walk fashion.

Stretch

Day 19

Strength Circuit

Warm Up
Gentle jog 5 mins (on the spot or on the move)
Mobilisation of joints – shoulder circles etc
30 jumping jacks
30 high knees
30 heel flicks
30 seconds jog on spot
5 second sprint on spot
Lying side leg lift x 20 each leg
Glute bridge x 20

Squats 2 x 15 Dead lifts 2 x 10 Pull ups 2 x 10 Dips 2 x 10 Renegade row 2 x 10 (each side) Plank 2 x 50 seconds	Pick a weight that allows you to perform the target number of reps with good form stopping before failure

Stretch

Day 20

Rest day – must go for a gentle walk

Day 21

Hill repeats

Warm Up
Gentle jog 5 mins (on the spot or on the move)
Mobilisation of joints – shoulder circles etc
30 jumping jacks
30 high knees
30 heel flicks
30 seconds jog on spot
5 second sprint on spot
Lying side leg lift x 20 each leg
Glute bridge x 20

Once warm, run up a short hill and then walk down this is 1 set. Perform 6 sets at 100% effort.

Cool down with gentle jog / walk for 5 minutes

Stretch

Day 22

Circuit

Warm Up
Gentle jog 5 mins (on the spot or on the move)
Mobilisation of joints – shoulder circles etc
30 jumping jacks
30 high knees
30 heel flicks
30 seconds jog on spot

5 second sprint on spot
Lying side leg lift x 20 each leg
Glute bridge x 20

30 seconds work 30 seconds rest. Do as many repetitions of each exercise with good form in 30 seconds, take 30 seconds rest and then perform that exercise again before moving on to the next exercise (30 seconds rest).

Burpees 30s x 2
Press ups 30s x 2
Squats 30s x 2
Pull ups 30s x 2
Alternate split squats 30s x 2
Shoulder press 30s x 2
Body row 30s x 2
Plank 30s x 2

Take 1 minute rest and then repeat.

Stretch

Day 23

Rest – must go for a walk and perform mobility exercises (as per warm ups)

Day 24

Rest – Must go for a walk and perform mobility exercises (as per warm ups)

Day 25

Test
Aerobic Fitness Test. This is a 12 minute test to measure the efficiency of your circulatory and respiratory system in supplying oxygen to your muscles during physical activity.

Spend 15 minutes warming up and then run as far as you can for 12 minutes. You will need to be able to track the distance you are running. This test is ideally performed on a running track, however a treadmill can be used (1% gradient must be applied).

Test Results

Male

Age	Excellent	Above Average	Average	Below Average	Poor
17-19	>3000m	2700-3000m	2500-2699m	2300-2499m	<2300m
20-29	>2800m	2400-2800m	2200-2399m	1600-2199m	<1600m
30-39	>2700m	2300-2700m	1900-2299m	1500-1899m	<1500m
40-49	>2500m	2100-2500m	1700-2099m	1400-1699m	<1400m
>50	>2400m	2000-2400m	1600-1999m	1300-1599m	<1300m

Female

Age	Excellent	Above Average	Average	Below Average	Poor
17-19	>2300m	2100-2300m	1800-2099m	1700-1799m	<1700m
20-29	>2700m	2200-2700m	1800-2199m	1500-1799m	<1500m
30-39	>2500m	2000-2500m	1700-1999m	1400-1699m	<1400m
40-49	>2300m	1900-2300m	1500-1899m	1200-1499m	<1200m
>50	>2200m	1700-2200m	1400-1699m	1100-1399m	<1100m

Muscular Fitness Test (2 second timer applied to press up test)

Exercise	Excellent	Above Average	Average	Below Average	Poor
Press Ups	>60	40-60	25-39	10 – 24	<10
Pull Ups	>16	11 – 16	7 – 10	3 – 6	<2
Plank	>4:00	3:01 – 4:00	2:01 – 3:00	1:00 – 2:00	<1:00

Test	Your Score	Date	Target for next test
Cooper Test			
Press Ups			
Pull Ups			
Plank			

Review:

Check your results, this test should highlight your strengths and weaknesses and what has improved / not improved.

Day 26

Run

Warm Up
Gentle jog 5 mins (on the spot or on the move)
Mobilisation of joints – shoulder circles etc
30 jumping jacks
30 high knees
30 heel flicks
30 seconds jog on spot
5 second sprint on spot
Lying side leg lift x 20 each leg
Glute bridge x 20

6Km run steady pace. If you cannot run the full distance complete in run/walk fashion.

Stretch

Day 27

Strength Circuit

Warm Up
Gentle jog 5 mins (on the spot or on the move)
Mobilisation of joints – shoulder circles etc
30 jumping jacks
30 high knees
30 heel flicks
30 seconds jog on spot
5 second sprint on spot
Lying side leg lift x 20 each leg
Glute bridge x 20

Squats 3 x 15 Dead lifts 3 x 10 Pull ups 3 x 10 Dips 3 x 10 Renegade row 3 x 10 (each side) Plank 3 x 60 seconds	Pick a weight that allows you to perform the target number of reps with good form stopping before failure

Stretches

Day 28

Rest day – must go for a gentle walk

Day 29

Tempo Run

Warm Up
Gentle jog 5 mins (on the spot or on the move)
Mobilisation of joints – shoulder circles etc
30 jumping jacks
30 high knees
30 heel flicks
30 seconds jog on spot
5 second sprint on spot
Lying side leg lift x 20 each leg
Glute bridge x 20

Start running for 20 minutes at a steady pace
Increase speed for 20 minutes and maintain a fast pace that you can barely hold a conversation for. A good indicator is – if you can only say a few words at a time you are in the right zone.
After 20 minutes, reduce speed and run at a slow pace for 20 minutes and then begin cool down.
Stretch

Day 30

Circuit
Warm Up
Gentle jog 5 mins (on the spot or on the move)
Mobilisation of joints – shoulder circles etc
30 jumping jacks
30 high knees
30 heel flicks
30 seconds jog on spot
5 second sprint on spot
Lying side leg lift x 20 each leg
Glute bridge x 20

40 seconds work **20** seconds rest. Do as many repetitions of each exercise with good form in **40** seconds, take **20** seconds rest and then perform that exercise again before moving on to the next exercise (**20** seconds rest).

Burpees 40s x 2
Press ups 40s x 2
Squats 40s x 2

Pull ups 40s x 2
Alternate split squats 40s x 2
Shoulder press 40s x 2
Body row 40s x 2
Plank 40s x 2

Take 1 minute rest and then repeat.
Stretch

Day 31

<u>Run</u>
Warm Up
Slow Steady Run 5.5km
Stretch

Day 32

<u>**Intensity Circuit**</u>

Warm Up
Lying side leg lift x 30 each leg
Glute bridge x 30

Set a timer for 15 minutes. Complete as many rounds as possible of the following circuits in 15 minutes (exercises must be done with good form).

Burpees x 15
Squat jumps x 15
Squat thrusts x 15
Press ups x 15

Excellent	Above Average	Average	Below Average	Poor
8 or more	5 – 7	4 – 5	2 – 3	<2

2 Minute rest

Sprints
You will require a set distance of 50 metres for this section.
Perform 6 shuttle runs of 50 metres at 50% effort
Perform 6 x shuttles sprints of 50 metres at 100% effort (rest period is a slow 50 metre return jog)

2 Minute rest

(continued on next page)

Superset
Perform each exercise one after the other for 3 rounds

Pull ups – as many as possible (with good form
Plank – 60 seconds

Stretch

Day 33

Rest – Active recovery

Day 34

Loaded March
Warm Up
For this section you will require suitable walking boots and a ruck sack. Put 5 Kg of weight in the rucksack. If you are using water bottles remember that 1 Litre = 1 Kg.
Other suggestions could be weights, fishing weights, sand, books, etc. Ensure that there is a comfortable fit and suitable padding to prevent anything from rubbing on your back.
Distance: Once warm, walk 3 Miles. Ideally up hill, even if this means repeatedly walking up and down a small hill! Do not run.

Stretch

Day 35

Circuit
Warm Up
Gentle jog 5 mins (on the spot or on the move)
Mobilisation of joints – shoulder circles etc
30 jumping jacks, 30 high knees
30 heel flicks, 30 seconds jog on spot
5 second sprint on spot
Lying side leg lift x 20 each leg
Glute bridge x 20

40 seconds work **20** seconds rest. Do as many repetitions of each exercise with good form in **40** seconds, take **20** seconds rest and then perform that exercise again before moving on to the next exercise (**20** seconds rest).

Burpees 40s x 2
Press ups 40s x 2
Squats 40s x 2
Pull ups 40s x 2

Alternate split squats 40s x 2
Shoulder press 40s x 2
Body row 40s x 2
Plank 40s x 2

Take 1 minute rest and then repeat.
Stretch

Day 36

Run

Warm Up
Run 6 Km at a steady pace

Stretch

Day 37

Rest – Ensure you keep moving, go for a walk and do mobilisation drills.

Day 38

Tempo Run

Warm Up
Start running for 20 minutes at a steady pace
Increase speed for 20 minutes and maintain a fast pace that you can barely hold a conversation for. A good indicator is – if you can only say a few words at a time you are in the right zone.
After 20 minutes, reduce speed and run at a slow pace for 20 minutes and then begin cool down.

Stretch

Day 39

Circuit

Warm Up
Gentle jog 5 mins (on the spot or on the move)
Mobilisation of joints – shoulder circles etc
30 jumping jacks
30 high knees
30 heel flicks
30 seconds jog on spot
5 second sprint on spot
Lying side leg lift x 20 each leg
Glute bridge x 20

40 seconds work 20 seconds rest. Do as many repetitions of each exercise with good form in 40 seconds, take 20 seconds rest and then perform that exercise again before moving on to the next exercise (20 seconds rest).

Burpees 40s x 2
Press ups 40s x 2
Squats 40s x 2
Pull ups 40s x 2
Alternate split squats 40s x 2
Shoulder press 40s x 2
Body row 40s x 2
Plank 40s x 2

Take 1 minute rest and then repeat.

Stretch

Day 40

Run

Warm Up
Run 6.5 Km at a steady pace

Stretch

Day 41

Intensity Circuit

Warm Up
Lying side leg lift x 30 each leg
Glute bridge x 30

Set a timer for 15 minutes. Complete as many rounds as possible of the following circuits in 15 minutes (exercises must be done with good form).

Burpees x 15
Squat jumps x 15
Squat thrusts x 15
Press ups x 15

Excellent	Above Average	Average	Below Average	Poor
8 or more	5 – 7	4 – 5	2 – 3	<2

2 Minute rest

Sprints
You will require a set distance of 50 metres for this section.
Perform 6 shuttle runs of 50 metres at 50% effort
Perform 6 x shuttles sprints of 50 metres at 100% effort (rest period is a slow 50 metre return jog)

2 Minute rest

Superset
Perform each exercise one after the other for 3 rounds

Pull ups – as many as possible with good form

Plank – 60 seconds

Stretch

Day 42 & 43

Rest

Day 44

Test

Aerobic Fitness Test. This is a 12 minute test to measure the efficiency of your circulatory and respiratory system in supplying oxygen to your muscles during physical activity.

Spend 15 minutes warming up and then run as far as you can for 12 minutes. You will need to be able to track the distance you are running. This test is ideally performed on a running track, however a treadmill can be used (1% gradient must be applied).

Test Results

Male

Age	Excellent	Above Average	Average	Below Average	Poor
17-19	>3000m	2700-3000m	2500-2699m	2300-2499m	<2300m
20-29	>2800m	2400-2800m	2200-2399m	1600-2199m	<1600m
30-39	>2700m	2300-2700m	1900-2299m	1500-1899m	<1500m
40-49	>2500m	2100-2500m	1700-2099m	1400-1699m	<1400m
>50	>2400m	2000-2400m	1600-1999m	1300-1599m	<1300m

Female

Age	Excellent	Above Average	Average	Below Average	Poor
17-19	>2300m	2100-2300m	1800-2099m	1700-1799m	<1700m
20-29	>2700m	2200-2700m	1800-2199m	1500-1799m	<1500m
30-39	>2500m	2000-2500m	1700-1999m	1400-1699m	<1400m
40-49	>2300m	1900-2300m	1500-1899m	1200-1499m	<1200m
>50	>2200m	1700-2200m	1400-1699m	1100-1399m	<1100m

Muscular Fitness Test (2 minute timer applies for press ups)

Exercise	Excellent	Above Average	Average	Below Average	Poor
Press Ups	>60	40-60	25-39	10 – 24	<10
Pull Ups	>16	11 – 16	7 – 10	3 – 6	<2
Plank	>4:00	3:01 – 4:00	2:01 – 3:00	1:00 – 2:00	<1:00

Test	Your Score	Date	Target for next test
Cooper Test			
Press Ups			
Pull Ups			
Plank			

Review:

Check your results, this test should highlight your strengths and weaknesses and what has improved / not improved.

Day 45

Rest

Day 46

Run

Warm Up
Run 7 Km at a steady pace. **Stretch upon completion.**

Day 47

Circuit

Warm Up
Gentle jog 5 mins (on the spot or on the move)
Mobilisation of joints – shoulder circles etc
30 jumping jacks
30 high knees
30 heel flicks
30 seconds jog on spot
5 second sprint on spot
Lying side leg lift x 20 each leg
Glute bridge x 20

40 seconds work 20 seconds rest. Do as many repetitions of each exercise with good form in 40 seconds, take 20 seconds rest and then perform that exercise again before moving on to the next exercise (20 seconds rest).

Burpees 40s x 2
Press ups 40s x 2
Squats 40s x 2
Pull ups 40s x 2
Alternate split squats 40s x 2
Shoulder press 40s x 2
Body row 40s x 2
Plank 40s x 2

Take 1 minute rest and then repeat. **Stretch upon completion.**

Day 48

Loaded March

Warm Up
For this section you will require suitable walking boots and a ruck sack. Put 5 Kg of weight in the rucksack. If you are using water bottles remember that 1 Litre = 1 Kg.

Other suggestions could be weights, fishing weights, sand, books, etc. Ensure that there is a comfortable fit and suitable padding to prevent anything from rubbing on your back.
Distance: Once warm, walk 3 Miles. Ideally up hill, even if this means repeatedly walking up and down a small hill! Do not run.

Stretch

Day 49

Rest

Day 50

Run

Warm Up
Run 7.5 Km at a steady pace

Stretch

Day 51

Intensity Circuit

Warm Up
Lying side leg lift x 30 each leg
Glute bridge x 30

Set a timer for 15 minutes. Complete as many rounds as possible of the following circuits in 15 minutes (exercises must be done with good form).

Burpees x 15
Squat jumps x 15
Squat thrusts x 15
Press ups x 15

Excellent	Above Average	Average	Below Average	Poor
8 or more	5 – 7	4 – 5	2 – 3	<2

2 Minute rest

Sprints
You will require a set distance of 50 metres for this section.
Perform 6 shuttle runs of 50 metres at 50% effort
Perform 6 x shuttles sprints of 50 metres at 100% effort (rest period is a slow 50 metre return jog)

2 Minute rest

Superset
Perform each exercise one after the other for 3 rounds

Pull ups – as many as possible with good form

Plank – 60 seconds

Stretch

Day 52

Loaded March

Warm Up
For this section you will require suitable walking boots and a ruck sack. Put 5 Kg of weight in the rucksack. If you are using water bottles remember that 1 Litre = 1 Kg.

Other suggestions could be weights, fishing weights, sand, books, etc. Ensure that there is a comfortable fit and suitable padding to prevent anything from rubbing on your back.
Distance: Once warm, walk 3 Miles. Ideally up hill, even if this means repeatedly walking up and down a small hill! Do not run.

Stretch

Day 53

Rest

Day 54

Run

Warm Up
Run 7 Km at a steady pace

Stretch

Day 55

Circuit

Warm Up
Gentle jog 5 mins (on the spot or on the move)
Mobilisation of joints – shoulder circles etc
30 jumping jacks
30 high knees
30 heel flicks
30 seconds jog on spot
5 second sprint on spot
Lying side leg lift x 20 each leg
Glute bridge x 20

50 seconds work **10** seconds rest. Do as many repetitions of each exercise with good form in **50** seconds, take **10** seconds rest and then perform that exercise again before moving on to the next exercise (**10** seconds rest).

Burpees 50s x 2
Press ups 50s x 2
Squats 50s x 2
Pull ups 50s x 2
Alternate split squats 50s x 2
Shoulder press 50s x 2
Body row 50s x 2
Plank 50s x 2

Take 1 minute rest and then repeat.

Stretch

Day 56

Hill repeats

Warm Up (20 minutes)
Once warm, run up a short hill and then walk down this is 1 set. Perform 8 sets at 100% effort.

Cool down with gentle jog / walk for 5 minutes

Stretch

Day 57

Rest

Day 58

Run

Warm Up
Run 7.5 Km at a steady pace

Stretch

Day 59

Intensity Circuit
Warm Up
Lying side leg lift x 30 each leg
Glute bridge x 30
Set a timer for 15 minutes. Complete as many rounds as possible of the following circuits in 15 minutes (exercises must be done with good form).
Burpees x 15
Squat jumps x 15
Squat thrusts x 15
Press ups x 15

Excellent	Above Average	Average	Below Average	Poor
8 or more	5 – 7	4 – 5	2 – 3	<2

2 Minute rest
Sprints
You will require a set distance of 50 metres for this section.
Perform 6 shuttle runs of 50 metres at 50% effort
Perform 6 x shuttles sprints of 50 metres at 100% effort (rest period is a slow 50 metre return jog)

2 Minute rest
Superset
Perform each exercise one after the other for 3 rounds
Pull ups – as many as possible with good form
Plank – 60 seconds

Stretch

Day 60

Loaded March

Warm Up
For this section you will require suitable walking boots and a ruck sack. Put **7 Kg** of weight in the rucksack. If you are using water bottles remember that 1 Litre = 1 Kg.

Other suggestions could be weights, fishing weights, sand, books, etc. Ensure that there is a comfortable fit and suitable padding to prevent anything from rubbing on your back.

Distance: Once warm, walk 3 Miles. Ideally up hill, even if this means repeatedly walking up and down a small hill! Do not run.

Stretch

Day 61

Rest

Day 62

Tempo Run

Warm Up
Start running for 20 minutes at a steady pace
Increase speed for 20 minutes and maintain a fast pace that you can barely hold a conversation for. A good indicator is – if you can only say a few words at a time you are in the right zone.
After 20 minutes, reduce speed and run at a slow pace for 20 minutes and then begin cool down.

Stretches

Day 63

Circuit

Warm Up
Gentle jog 5 mins (on the spot or on the move)
Mobilisation of joints – shoulder circles etc
40 jumping jacks
40 high knees
30 heel flicks
30 seconds jog on spot
5 second sprint on spot
Lying side leg lift x 30 each leg
Glute bridge x 30

50 seconds work 10 seconds rest. Do as many repetitions of each exercise with good form in 50 seconds, take 10 seconds rest and then perform that exercise again before moving on to the next exercise (10 seconds rest).

Burpees 50s x 2
Press ups 50s x 2
Squats 50s x 2
Pull ups 50s x 2
Alternate split squats 50s x 2
Shoulder press 50s x 2
Body row 50s x 2
Plank 50s x 2

Take 1 minute rest and then repeat.

Stretches

Day 64

Hill repeats

Warm Up (20 minutes)

Once warm, run up a short hill and then walk down this is 1 set. Perform 8 sets at 100% effort.

Cool down with gentle jog / walk for 5 minutes

Stretch

Day 65

Rest

Day 66

Run
Warm Up
Run 8 Km at a steady pace. **Stretch upon completion.**

Day 67

Intensity Circuit

Warm Up
Lying side leg lift x 30 each leg
Glute bridge x 30

Set a timer for 15 minutes. Complete as many rounds as possible of the following circuits in 15 minutes (exercises must be done with good form).

Burpees x 15
Squat jumps x 15
Squat thrusts x 15
Press ups x 15

Excellent	Above Average	Average	Below Average	Poor
8 or more	5 – 7	4 – 5	2 – 3	<2

2 Minute rest

Sprints
You will require a set distance of 50 metres for this section.
Perform 6 shuttle runs of 50 metres at 50% effort
Perform 6 x shuttles sprints of 50 metres at 100% effort (rest period is a slow 50 metre return jog)

2 Minute rest

Superset
Perform each exercise one after the other for 3 rounds

Pull ups – as many as possible with good form

Plank – 60 seconds
Stretch

Day 68

Loaded March

Warm Up

For this section you will require suitable walking boots and a ruck sack. Put **8 Kg** of weight in the rucksack. If you are using water bottles remember that 1 Litre = 1 Kg.

Other suggestions could be weights, fishing weights, sand, books, etc. Ensure that there is a comfortable fit and suitable padding to prevent anything from rubbing on your back.

Distance: Once warm, walk 3 Miles. Ideally up hill, even if this means repeatedly walking up and down a small hill! Do not run.
Stretch

Day 69

Circuit

Warm Up
Gentle jog 5 mins (on the spot or on the move)
Mobilisation of joints – shoulder circles etc
40 jumping jacks
40 high knees
30 heel flicks
30 seconds jog on spot
5 second sprint on spot
Lying side leg lift x 30 each leg
Glute bridge x 30

50 seconds work 10 seconds rest. Do as many repetitions of each exercise with good form in 50 seconds, take 10 seconds rest and then perform that exercise again before moving on to the next exercise (10 seconds rest).

Burpees 50s x 2
Press ups 50s x 2
Squats 50s x 2
Pull ups 50s x 2
Alternate split squats 50s x 2
Shoulder press 50s x 2
Body row 50s x 2
Plank 50s x 2

Take 1 minute rest and then repeat.

Stretch

Day 70 & 71

Rest

Day 72

Test:
Aerobic Fitness Test. This is a 12 minute test to measure the efficiency of your circulatory and respiratory system in supplying oxygen to your muscles during physical activity.

Spend 15 minutes warming up and then run as far as you can for 12 minutes. You will need to be able to track the distance you are running. This test is ideally performed on a running track, however a treadmill can be used (1% gradient must be applied).

Test Results

Male

Age	Excellent	Above Average	Average	Below Average	Poor
17-19	>3000m	2700-3000m	2500-2699m	2300-2499m	<2300m
20-29	>2800m	2400-2800m	2200-2399m	1600-2199m	<1600m
30-39	>2700m	2300-2700m	1900-2299m	1500-1899m	<1500m
40-49	>2500m	2100-2500m	1700-2099m	1400-1699m	<1400m
>50	>2400m	2000-2400m	1600-1999m	1300-1599m	<1300m

Female

Age	Excellent (5)	Above Average (4)	Average (3)	Below Average (2)	Poor (1)
17-19	>2300m	2100-2300m	1800-2099m	1700-1799m	<1700m
20-29	>2700m	2200-2700m	1800-2199m	1500-1799m	<1500m
30-39	>2500m	2000-2500m	1700-1999m	1400-1699m	<1400m
40-49	>2300m	1900-2300m	1500-1899m	1200-1499m	<1200m
>50	>2200m	1700-2200m	1400-1699m	1100-1399m	<1100m

Muscular Fitness Test (2 minute timer on press ups)

Exercise	Excellent (5)	Above Average (4)	Average (3)	Below Average (2)	Poor (1)
Press Ups	>60	40-60	25-39	10 – 24	<10
Pull Ups	>16	11 – 16	7 – 10	3 – 6	<2
Plank	>4:00	3:01 – 4:00	2:01 – 3:00	1:00 – 2:00	<1:00

Test	Your Score	Date	Total Points
Cooper Test			
Press Ups			
Pull Ups			
Plank			

In brackets you will see numbers, these are the points associated with your score. Add all these up to reach your total points

For example:

Test	Your Score	Date	Points
Cooper Test	2134m	01/01/21	Above average: 4
Press Ups	50	01/01/21	Above average: 4
Pull Ups	7	01/01/21	Average: 3
Plank	04:35:00	01/01/21	Excellent: 5
		TOTAL:	16

Maximum score is 20 and you will need this score for later on in the programme.

4 – 9 = Level 1
10 – 15 = Level 2
16 – 20 = Level 3

Day 73

Run

Warm Up
Run **9 Km** at a steady pace

Stretch

Day 74

Circuit 3

Warm Up
Gentle jog 5 mins (on the spot or on the move)
Mobilisation of joints – shoulder circles etc
40 jumping jacks
40 high knees
30 heel flicks
30 seconds jog on spot
5 second sprint on spot
Lying side leg lift x 40 each leg
Glute bridge x 40
Circuit 3 is split into 3 levels. This is based on your previous fitness test scores:

Exercise	Level 1	Level 2	Level 3
Burpees	150	200	300
Pull Ups	50	80	100
Close Press Ups	100	150	200
Body Row	100	120	150
Hanging Leg Raises	60	80	100

Divide the numbers by 10 and perform the circuit 10 times to complete the total, taking minimal rest.

On completion of that circuit:
Complete a gentle run of 5-10 minutes

800 metre sprint 100% effort.

Targets

Level 1	3 Minutes 15 seconds
Level 2	2 Minutes 46 seconds
Level 3	Less than 2 minutes 45 seconds

Stretch

Day 75

Rest

Day 76

Loaded March

Warm Up

For this section you will require suitable walking boots and a ruck sack. Put **9 Kg** of weight in the rucksack. If you are using water bottles remember that 1 Litre = 1 Kg.

Other suggestions could be weights, fishing weights, sand, books, etc. Ensure that there is a comfortable fit and suitable padding to prevent anything from rubbing on your back.

Distance: Once warm, walk 3 Miles. Ideally up hill, even if this means repeatedly walking up and down a small hill! Do not run.

Stretch

Day 77

Tempo Run

Warm Up
Start running for 20 minutes at a steady pace
Increase speed for 20 minutes and maintain a fast pace that you can barely hold a conversation for. A good indicator is – if you can only say a few words at a time you are in the right zone.
After 20 minutes, reduce speed and run at a slow pace for 20 minutes.

Mini Circuit

10 Pull Ups	
20 Press Ups	X 3
Plank 60 seconds	

Stretch

Day 78

Rest

Day 79

Run

Warm Up
Run **9.5 Km** at a steady pace

Stretch

Day 80

Circuit 3

Warm Up
Gentle jog 5 mins (on the spot or on the move)
Mobilisation of joints – shoulder circles etc
40 jumping jacks
40 high knees
30 heel flicks
30 seconds jog on spot
5 second sprint on spot
Lying side leg lift x **50** each leg
Glute bridge x **50**
Circuit 3 is split into 3 levels. This is based on your previous fitness test scores:

Exercise	Level 1	Level 2	Level 3
Burpees	170	220	350
Pull Ups	60	90	110
Close Press Ups	110	170	220
Body Row	120	140	170
Hanging Leg Raises	70	90	110

Divide the numbers by 10 and perform the circuit 10 times to complete the total, taking minimal rest.

On completion of that circuit:
Complete a gentle run of 5-10 minutes

2 x 800 metre sprint 100% effort. (Rest 5 minutes between sprints).

Targets

Level 1	3 Minutes 15 seconds
Level 2	2 Minutes 46 seconds
Level 3	Less than 2 minutes 45 seconds

Stretch

Day 81

Rest

Day 82

Loaded March

Warm Up

For this section you will require suitable walking boots and a ruck sack. Put **10 Kg** of weight in the rucksack. If you are using water bottles remember that 1 Litre = 1 Kg.

Other suggestions could be weights, fishing weights, sand, books, etc. Ensure that there is a comfortable fit and suitable padding to prevent anything from rubbing on your back.

Distance: Once warm, walk 3 Miles. Ideally up hill, even if this means repeatedly walking up and down a small hill! Do not run.

Stretch

Day 83

Tempo Run + Mini Circuit

Warm Up
Start running for 20 minutes at a steady pace
Increase speed for 20 minutes and maintain a fast pace that you can barely hold a conversation for. A good indicator is – if you can only say a few words at a time you are in the right zone.
After 20 minutes, reduce speed and run at a slow pace for 20 minutes.

Mini Circuit

10 Pull Ups	
20 Press Ups	X 3
Plank 60 seconds	

Stretch

Day 84

Rest

Day 85

Run + Mini Circuit

Warm Up
Run **10 Km** at a steady pace
Mini Circuit

10 Pull Ups	
20 Press Ups	X 3
Plank 60 seconds	

Stretch

Day 86

Rest

Day 87

Circuit 3

Warm Up
Gentle jog 5 mins (on the spot or on the move)
Mobilisation of joints – shoulder circles etc
40 jumping jacks
40 high knees
30 heel flicks
30 seconds jog on spot
5 second sprint on spot
Lying side leg lift x **50** each leg
Glute bridge x **50**
Circuit 3 is split into 3 levels. This is based on your previous fitness test scores:

Exercise	Level 1	Level 2	Level 3
Burpees	180	250	400
Pull Ups	70	100	120
Close Press Ups	110	180	230
Body Row	120	150	180
Hanging Leg Raises	80	100	120

Divide the numbers by 10 and perform the circuit 10 times to complete the total, taking minimal rest.

On completion of that circuit: *(next page)*

Complete a gentle run of 5-10 minutes

3 x 800 metre sprint 100% effort. (Rest 5 minutes between sprints).

Targets

Level 1	3 Minutes 15 seconds
Level 2	2 Minutes 46 seconds
Level 3	Less than 2 minutes 45 seconds

Stretch

Day 88 & 89

Rest

Day 90

Final Test

You have come a long way and worked hard to reach this point. Before you go into this test, think about those dark hard sessions where you had to dig deep, remember what you went through. It's time to prove it to yourself that you can go the distance and get results that you can be proud of.

Test:
Aerobic Fitness Test. This is a 12 minute test to measure the efficiency of your circulatory and respiratory system in supplying oxygen to your muscles during physical activity.

Spend 15 minutes warming up and then run as far as you can for 12 minutes. You will need to be able to track the distance you are running. This test is ideally performed on a running track, however a treadmill can be used (1% gradient must be applied).

Test Results

Male

Age	Excellent	Above Average	Average	Below Average	Poor
17-19	>3000m	2700-3000m	2500-2699m	2300-2499m	<2300m
20-29	>2800m	2400-2800m	2200-2399m	1600-2199m	<1600m
30-39	>2700m	2300-2700m	1900-2299m	1500-1899m	<1500m
40-49	>2500m	2100-2500m	1700-2099m	1400-1699m	<1400m
>50	>2400m	2000-2400m	1600-1999m	1300-1599m	<1300m

Female

Age	Excellent (5)	Above Average (4)	Average (3)	Below Average (2)	Poor (1)
17-19	>2300m	2100-2300m	1800-2099m	1700-1799m	<1700m
20-29	>2700m	2200-2700m	1800-2199m	1500-1799m	<1500m
30-39	>2500m	2000-2500m	1700-1999m	1400-1699m	<1400m
40-49	>2300m	1900-2300m	1500-1899m	1200-1499m	<1200m
>50	>2200m	1700-2200m	1400-1699m	1100-1399m	<1100m

Muscular Fitness Test

Exercise	Excellent (5)	Above Average (4)	Average (3)	Below Average (2)	Poor (1)
Press Ups	>60	40-60	25-39	10 – 24	<10
Pull Ups	>16	11 – 16	7 – 10	3 – 6	<2
Plank	>4:00	3:01 – 4:00	2:01 – 3:00	1:00 – 2:00	<1:00

Test	Your Score	Date	Total Points
Cooper Test			
Press Ups			
Pull Ups			
Plank			

Take a moment to compare you scores from day 1 to day 90

Well done for completing the programme, I hope you feel fitter and stronger than ever. Thank you so much for taking part in the Commando90 Series.

Exercise Guide

For Video Demonstrations please check the Commando90 Playlist on Muscle World Youtube channel:
https://youtube.com/playlist?list=PLkLVtk9NHtxV6lOe3lLR7EDGGr8u8Sv-G

High Knees

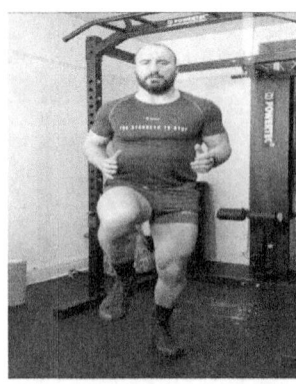

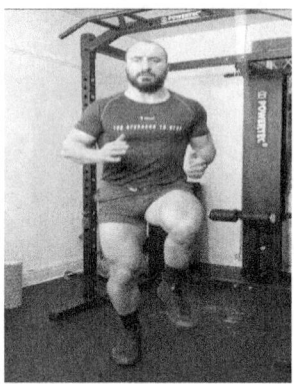

Jog on the spot and gradually lift your knees up, alternating your legs
Keep your core engaged, aim to lift your knees high enough so that your hips are parallel to the floor

Press Ups

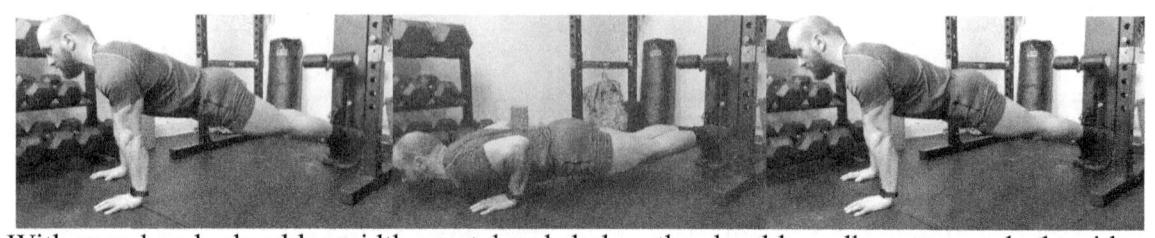

With your hands shoulder width apart, hands below the shoulders elbows towards the sides
1. Lower your chest to the floor, pivoting at the heel
2. Keep your body tight throughout
3. Full extend your arms

Press Ups with Knees Down

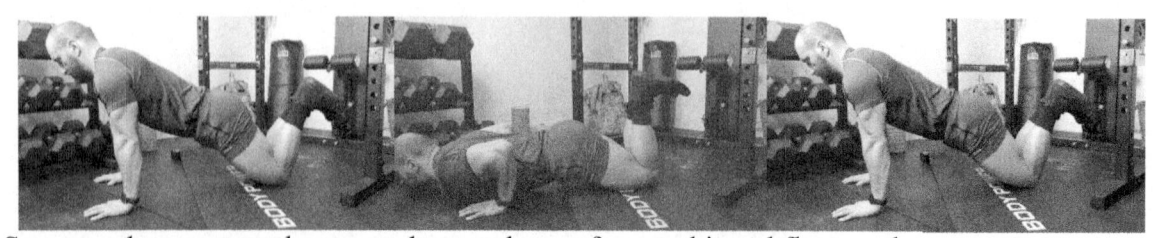

Same as above except knees are bent and on soft or cushioned floor such as a mat
1. Ensure the hips are forward of the knee

Close Press Ups

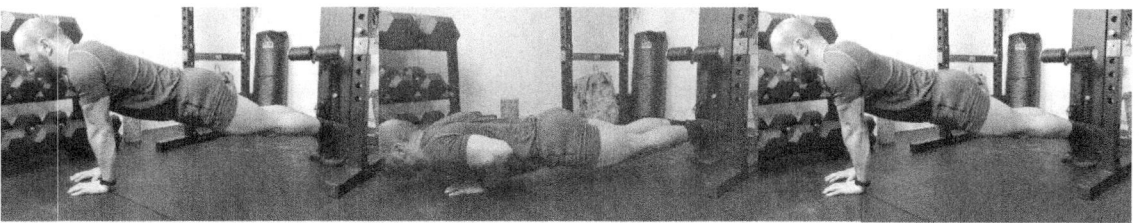

Same as press up except hands are brought close together

Shoulder Press With Ball

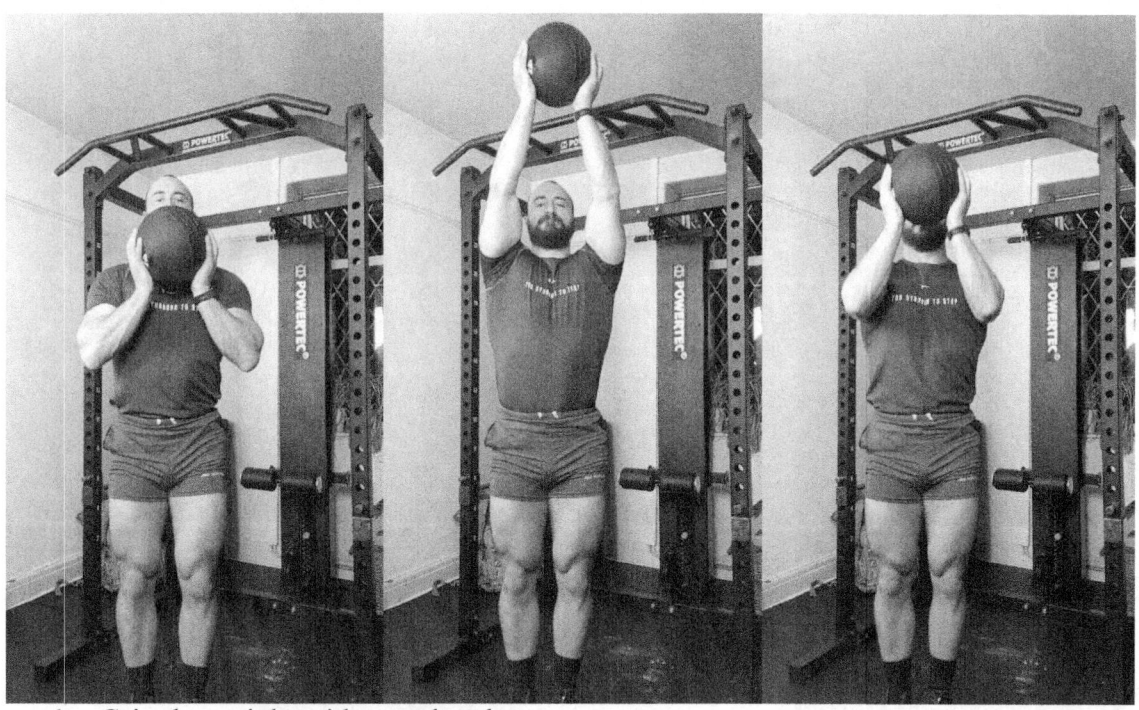

1. Grip the weight with your hands
2. Keep your core tight and tense your quads and glutes to create a strong platform
3. Extend your arms overhead
4. Slowly lower your arms back down so the weight is in front of your face
5. Repeat for desired number of repetitions

Shoulder Press With Dumbbells

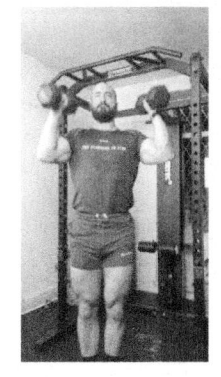

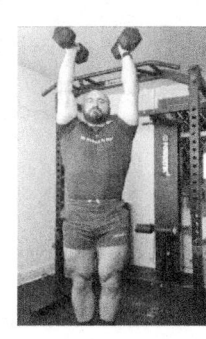

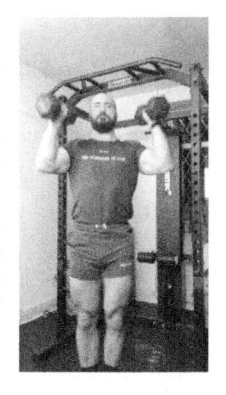

Body Row with Rope

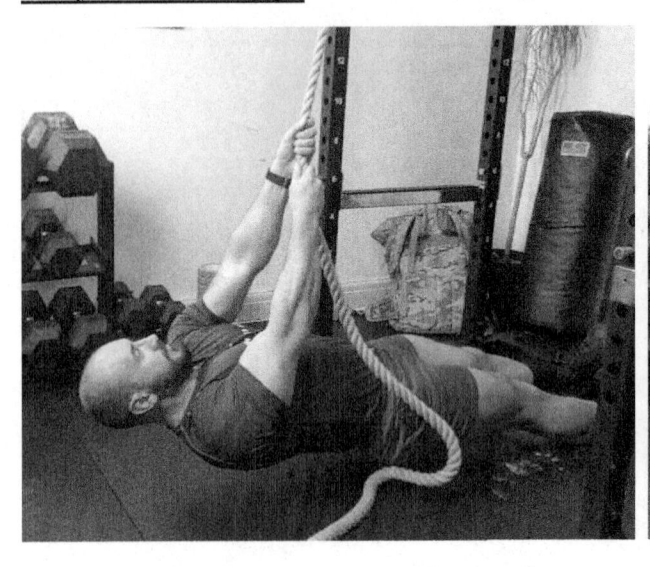

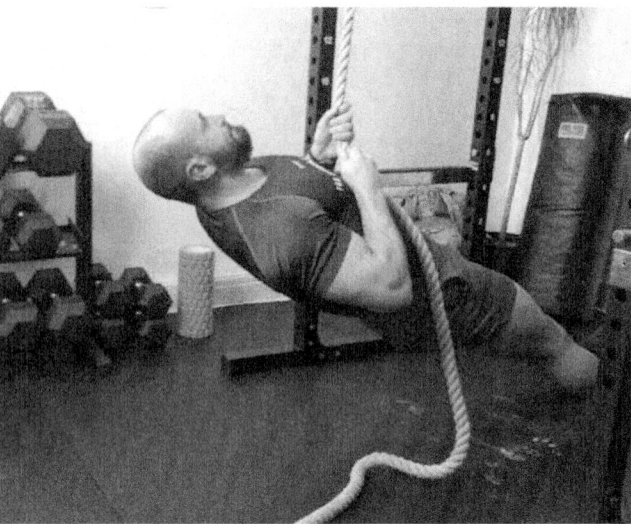

Body Row

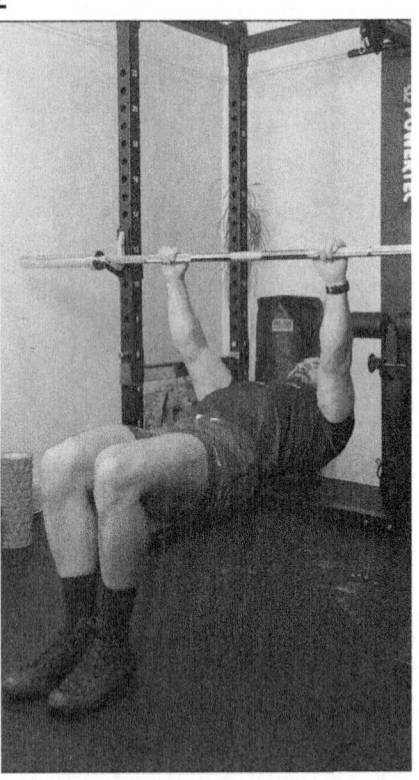

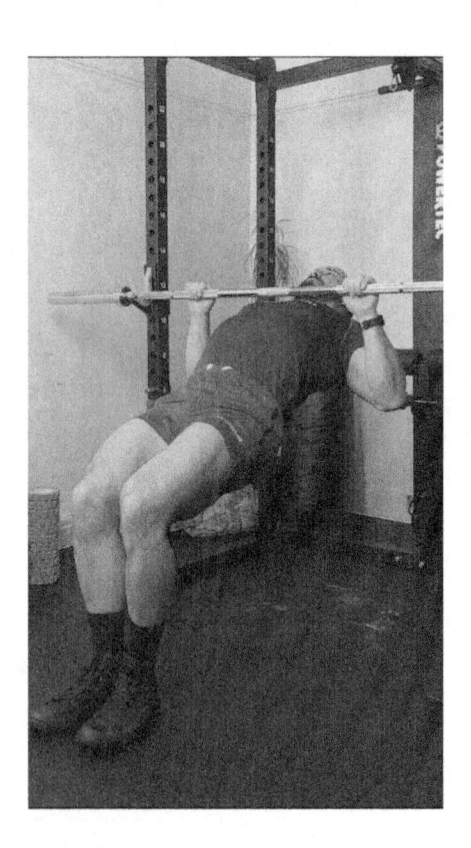

Ensure the equipment you are using is sturdy so that you will not fall.

1. Grip the rope / bar
2. Keeping your legs either straight
3. Pull yourself up keeping your core tight and engaged
4. Pivot at the feet
5. Slowly lower yourself down
6. Repeat for desired number of repetitions

Pull Ups

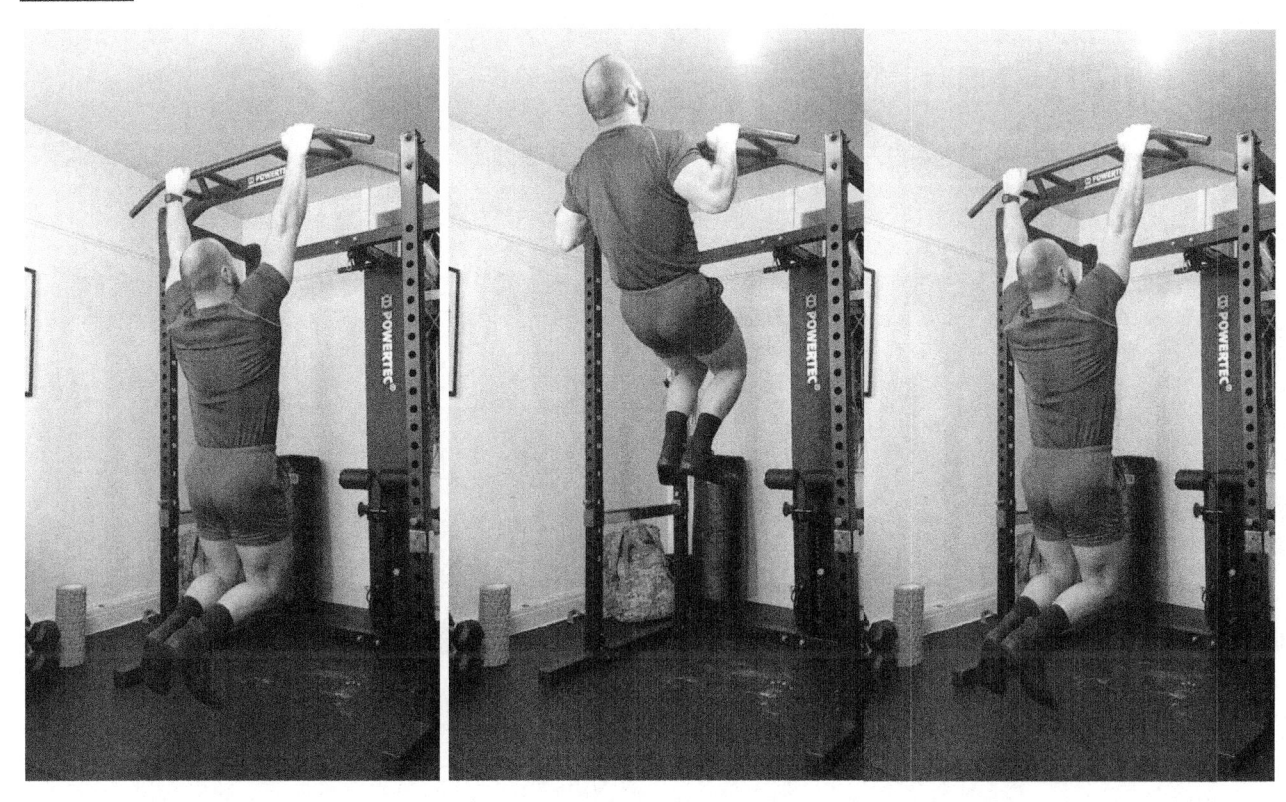

Pull Ups Assisted with Band (use if you cannot do 1 pull up. If you don't have a band jump or place feet on a bench to assist)

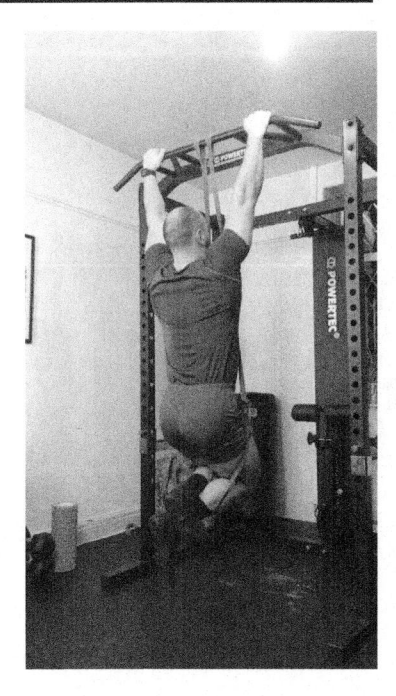

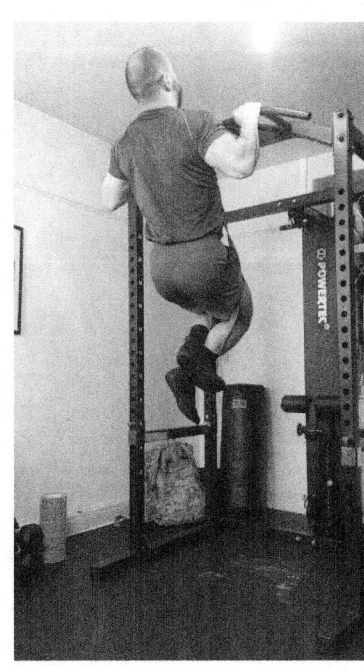

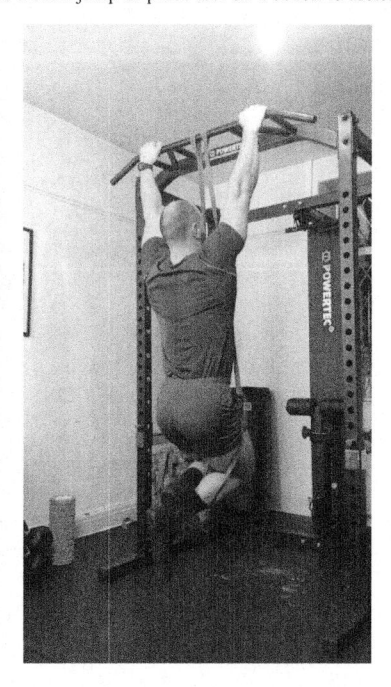

1. Use an overhand grip
2. Hang with arms straight
3. Without swinging pull your chest up to the bar
4. Slowly lower yourself down by straightening your arms
5. Repeat for desired number of repetitions

Burpee

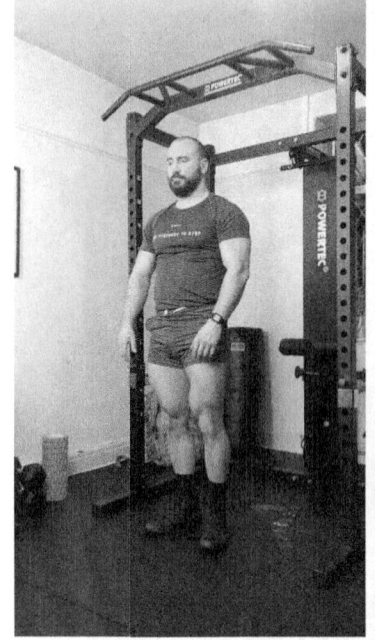

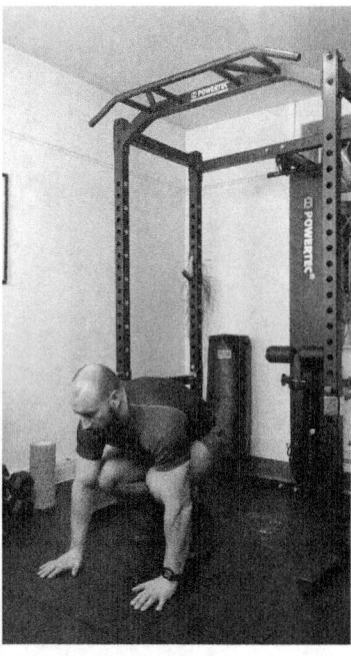

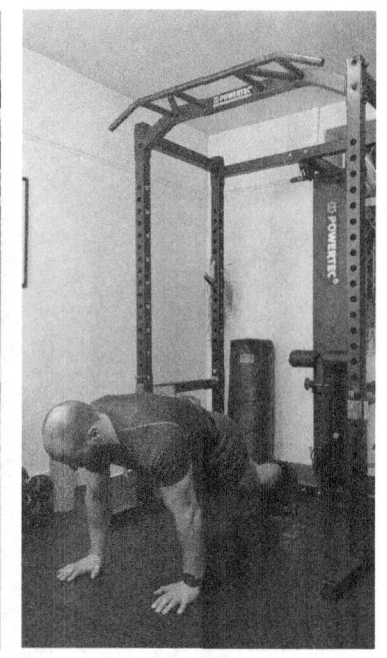

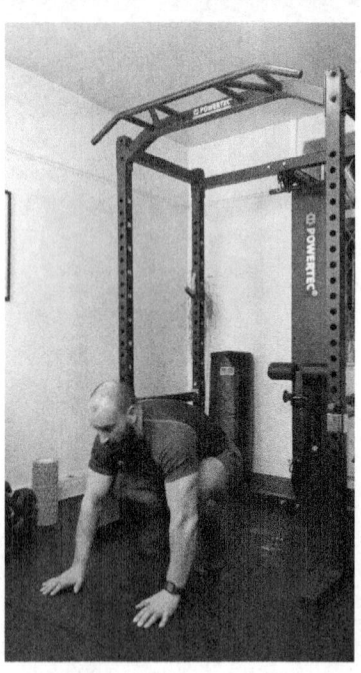

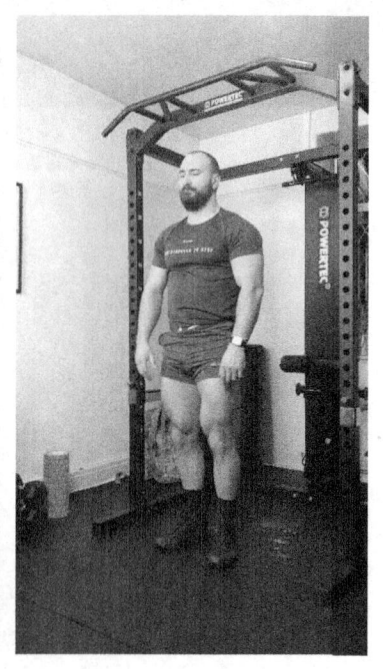

1. From a standing position bend at the knees bringing your hips towards the floor
2. Place your hands on the floor
3. Drive your legs back, full extending them
4. Keep your core engaged and tight throughout
5. Bring your knees back so you are in the squat position
6. Drive through the floor powerfully and extend your legs to return to the standing position
7. Repeat for desired number of repetitions

Squats

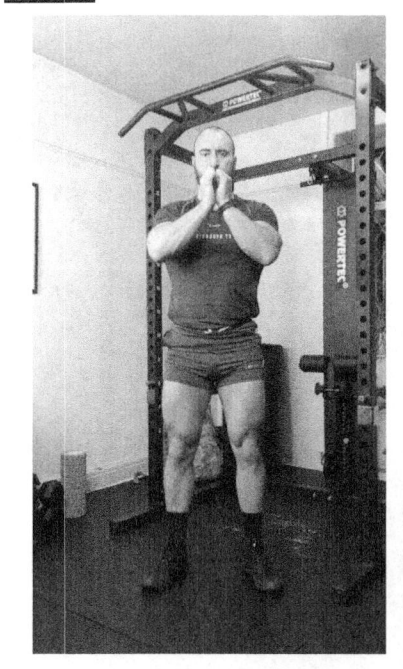

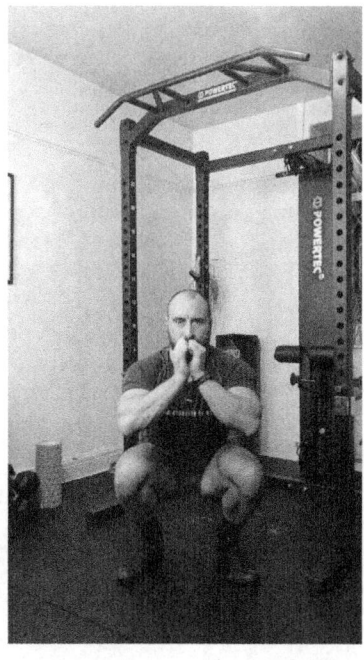

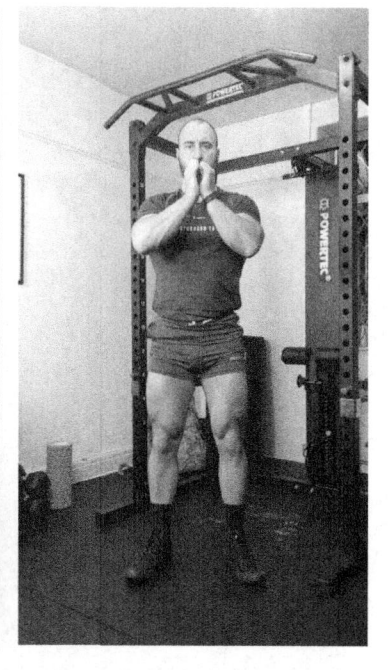

Stand tall with feet slightly wider than hip-width distance apart feet slightly turned out.

1. Look straight ahead and tighten your ab muscles
2. Bend your knees and sink your hips back while lowering your hips towards the floor. Try to keep a straight spine and tight core throughout the whole movement.
3. Straighten your legs and drive back up to standing position

Squats with dumbbell

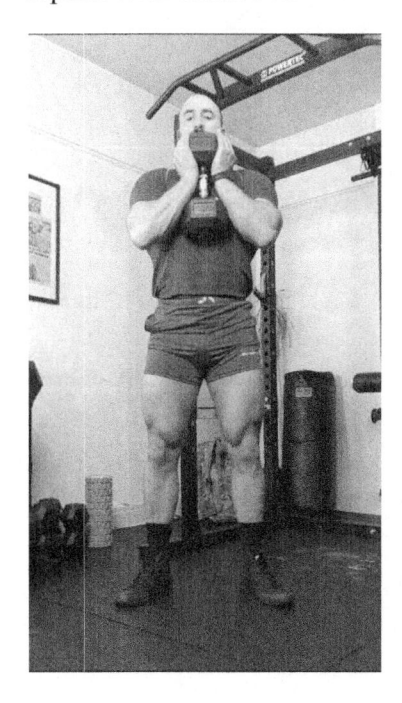

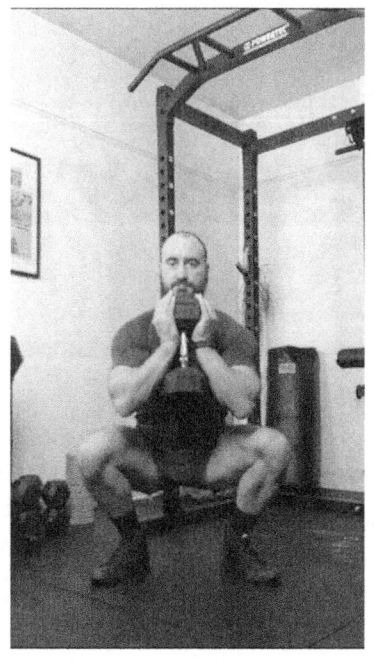

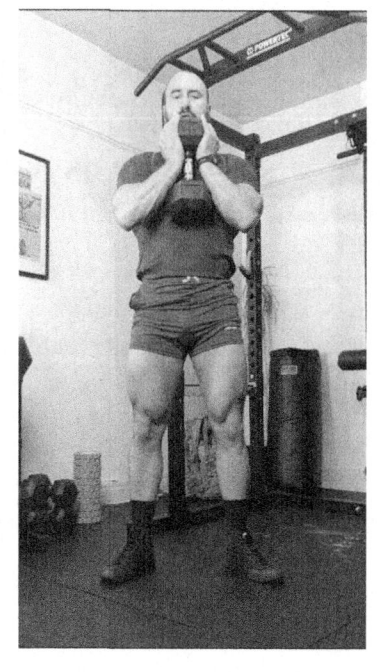

Squats with barbell

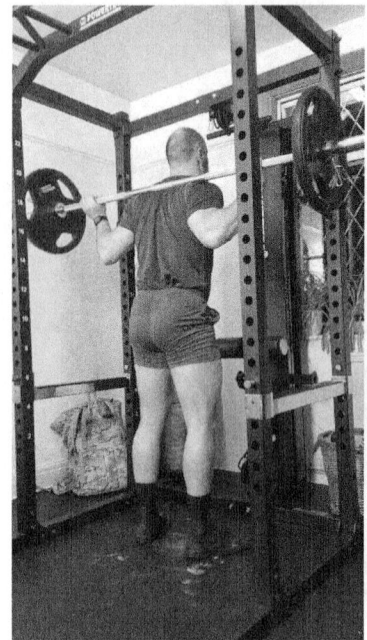

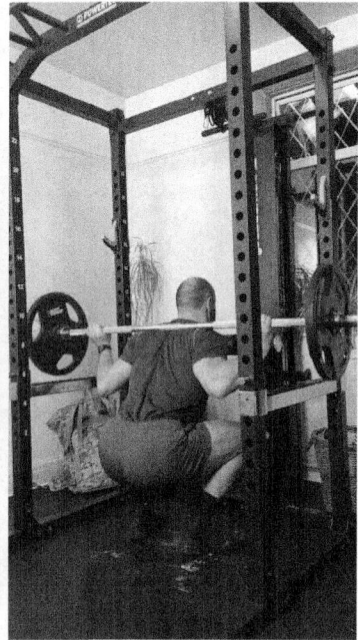

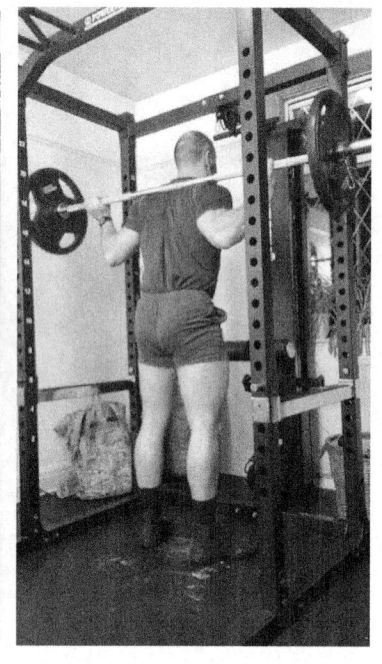

Alternating Split Squats

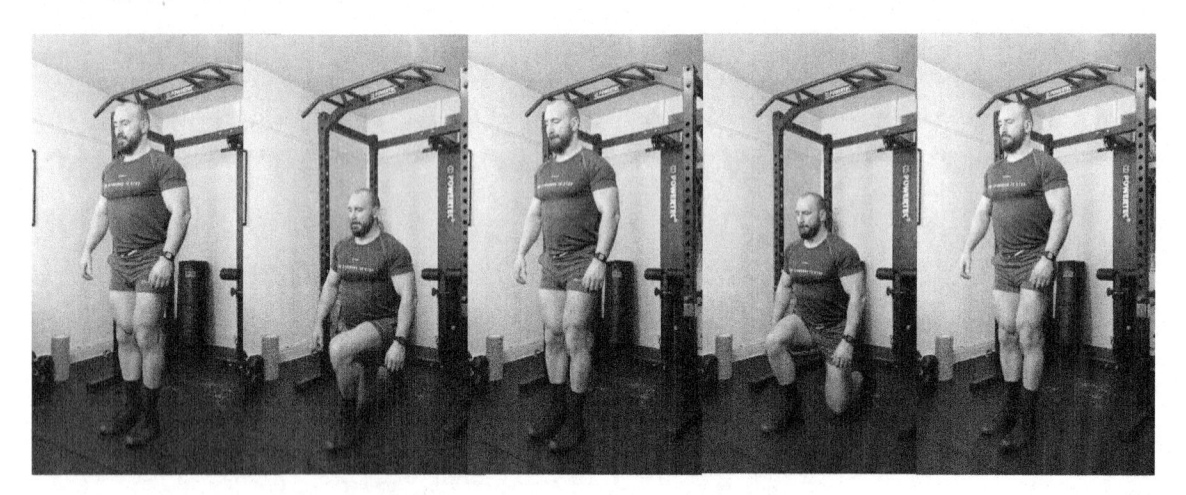

1. From the standing position step one leg back and bend at the knee slowly lowering your hips down towards the floor
2. Take care not to bang your knee on the floor!
3. Extend the front leg, stepping the rear leg forwards
4. Repeat on the opposite leg
5. Repeat process for desired number of repetitions

Plank

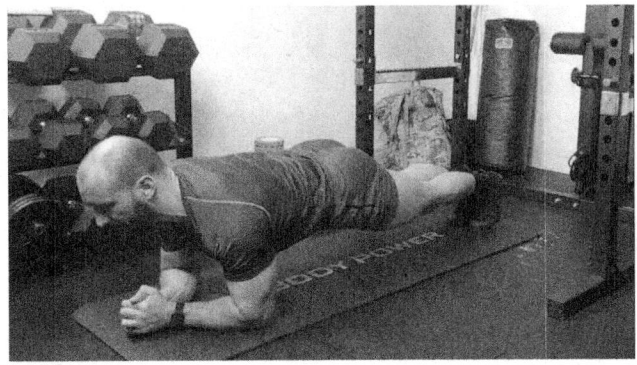

1. Elbows below the shoulder
2. Maintain a straight spine
3. Keep your core tight and engaged
4. Focus on your breathing

Squat Thrusts

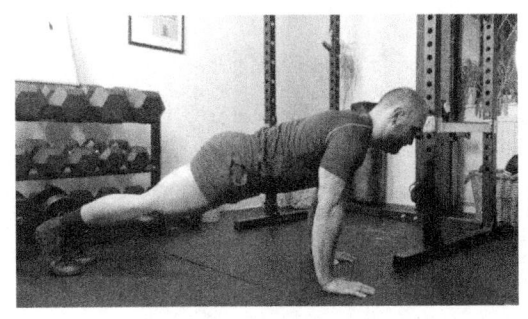

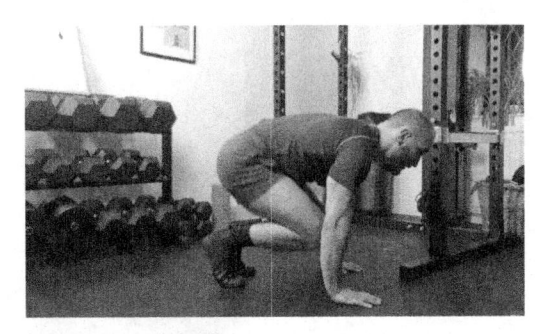

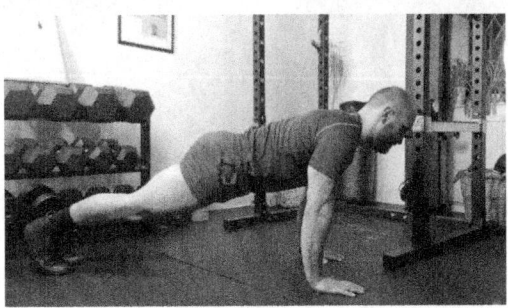

1. Start off in the press up position with your hands shoulder width apart and your hands below your shoulders.
2. Engage your core drive your knees under control towards your chest
3. Drive your legs backwards, fully extending your legs back to the starting positon
4. Keep your core braced through.

Lying Side Leg Lift

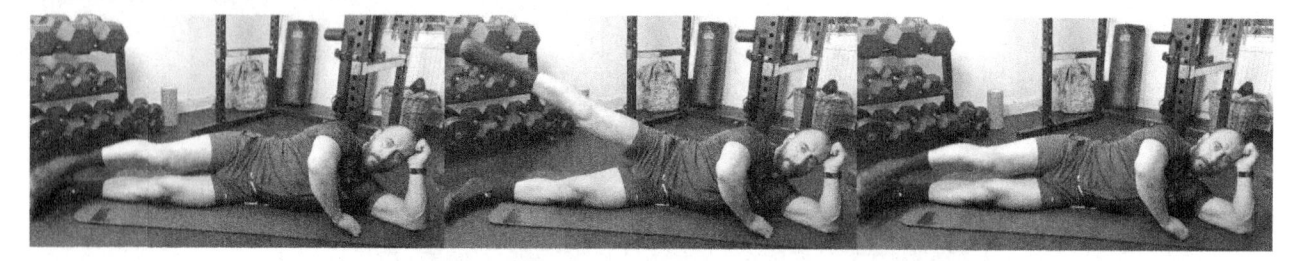

1. Lie on the side legs straight with your head supported by your hand
2. Slowly raise your top leg upwards, keep the side of your foot parallel to the floor
3. Slowly lower back down
4. Repeat for desired number of repetitions

Hanging Leg Raises

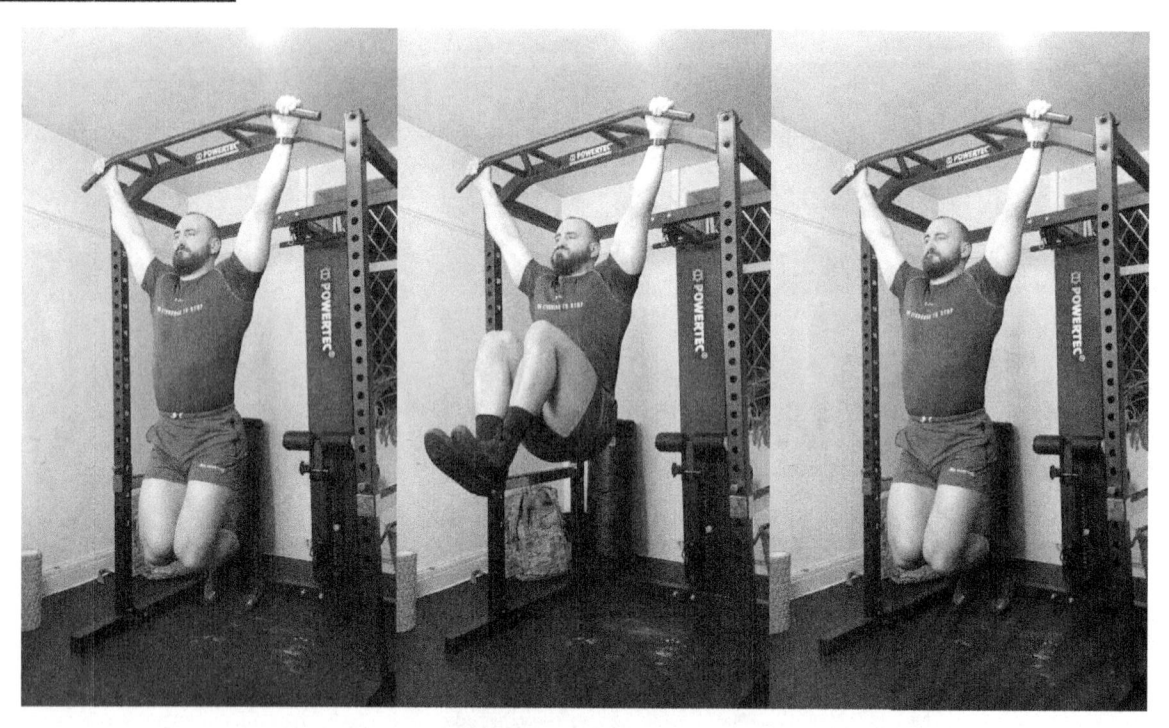

1. Hang from a suitable pull up bar with an overhand grip
2. Keeping your body stable engage your abs and hip flexors to raise your knees towards your chest
3. Slowly lower to the starting position
4. Repeat for desired number of repetitions, and remember this is a controlled movement without swinging

Hanging Leg Raises – with medicine ball squeeze

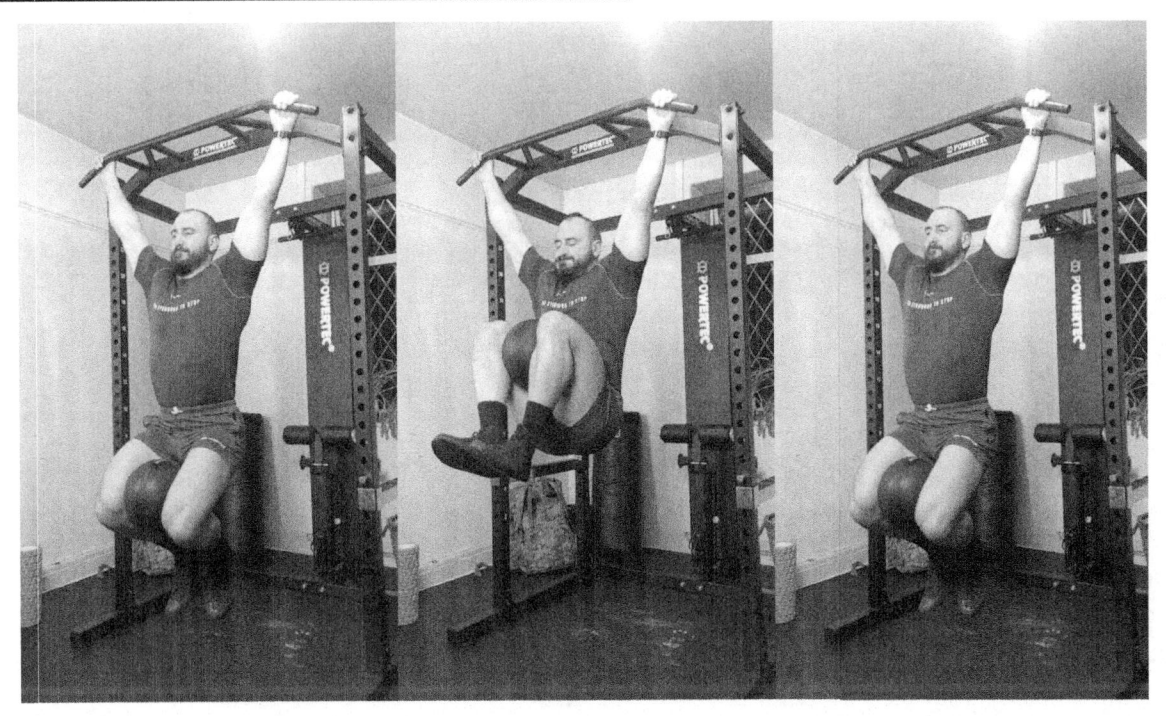

1. As above, except squeeze the medicine ball with your thighs to engage your adductor muscles
2. This is an excellent exercise for individuals in the military to assist with their rope climbing

Deadlift

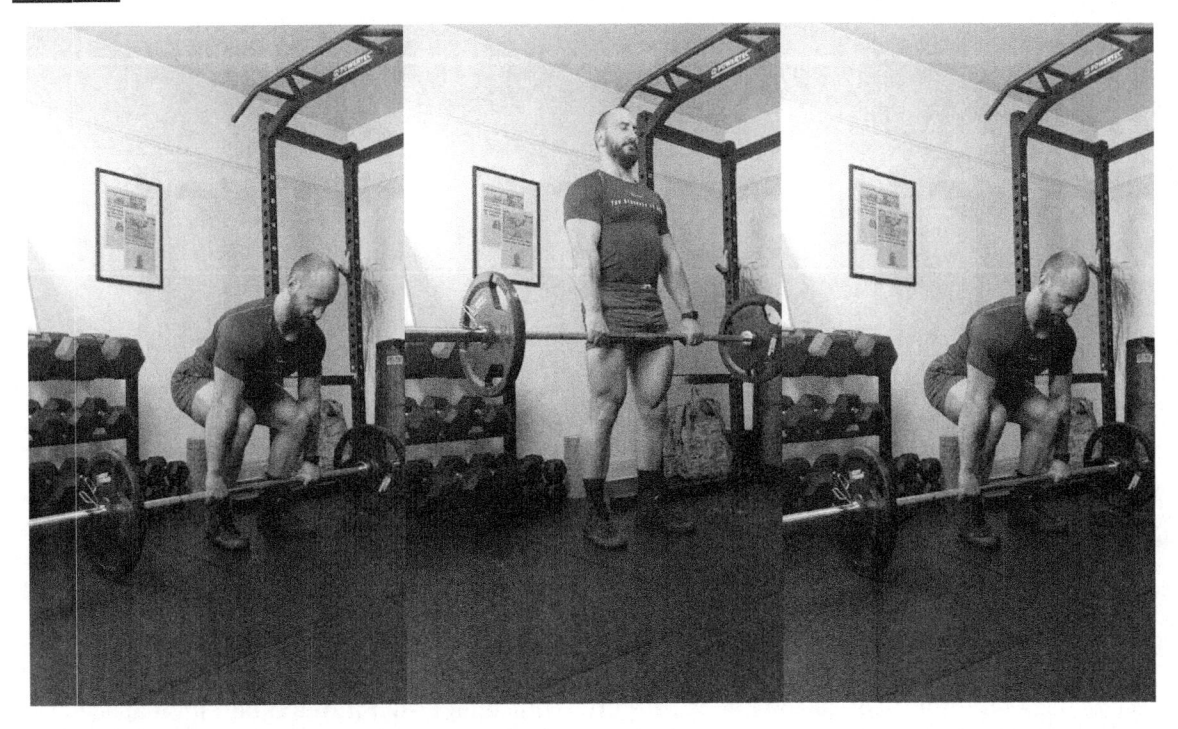

1. With feet shoulder width apart toes pointing forwards, grip the bar with an overhand grip
2. Keep your spine straight and drive through your feet extending at the knee and at the hip to stand up keeping the bar close to your body
3. Push your hips back and bend your knees to lower the bar back down to the floor

Jumping Jacks

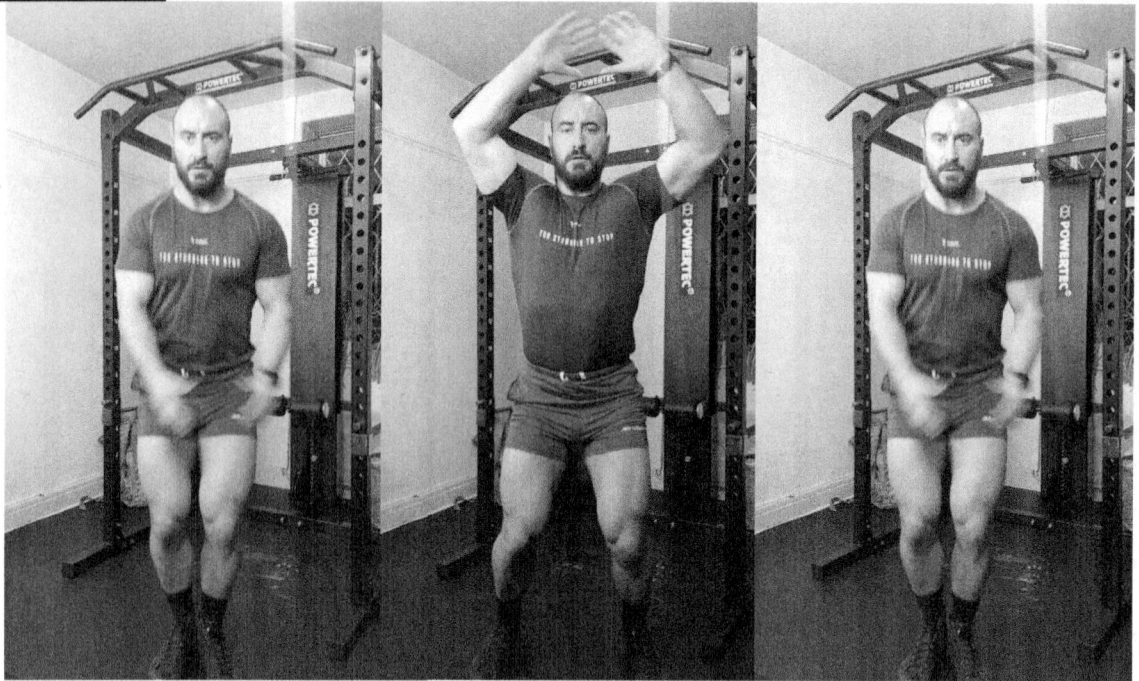

1. Stand upright with your legs together arms by the sides
2. Bend you knees slightly and jump into the air
3. As you jump spread your legs slightly to about shoulder width apart, lifting your arms up overhead
4. Ensure a nice soft landing with the knees and jump back to the starting position
5. Repeat for the desired number of repetitions.

Squat Jumps

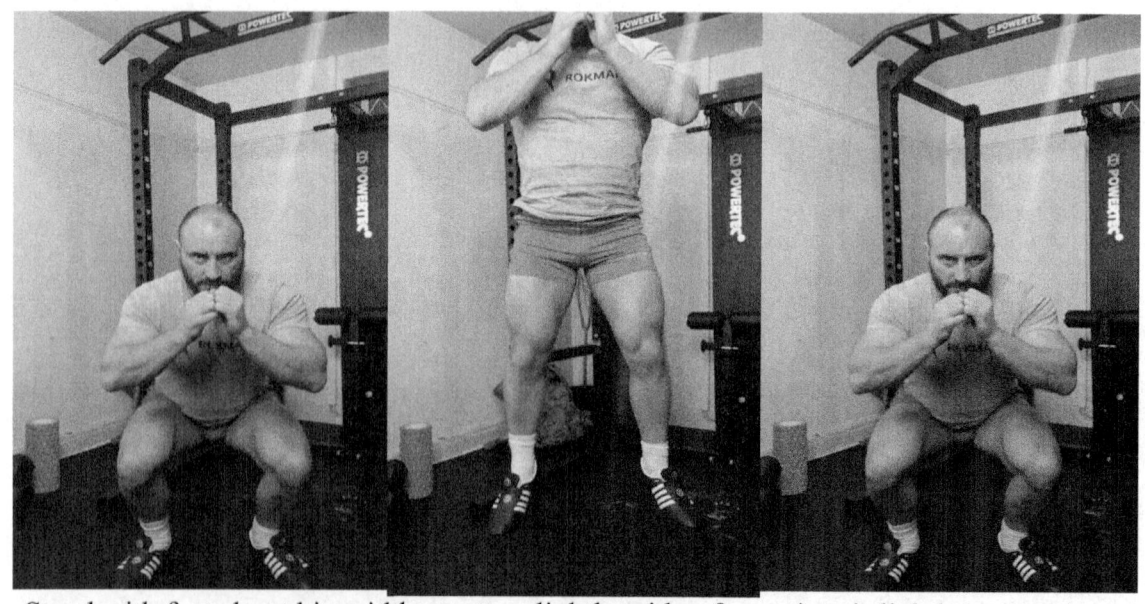

1. Stand with feet about hip width apart or slightly wider, feet pointed slightly outwards
2. Keeping your back straight, bend at the knees bringing your hips down into a quarter squat position (hips slightly above the knees)
3. Powerfully explode upwards into a jump
4. Land back down both feet at the same down sinking into a controlled descent
5. Repeat for desired number of repetitions

Glute Bridge

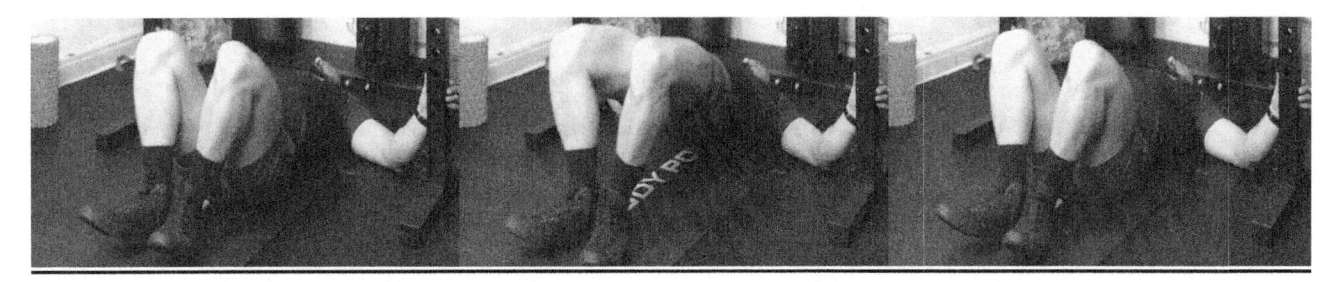

1. Lie down on the floor with knees bent and heels on the floor
2. Drive your heels in the ground and push your hips up
3. Pause for a second and tense your glutes
4. Slowly lower down to the starting position
5. Repeat for desired number of repetitions

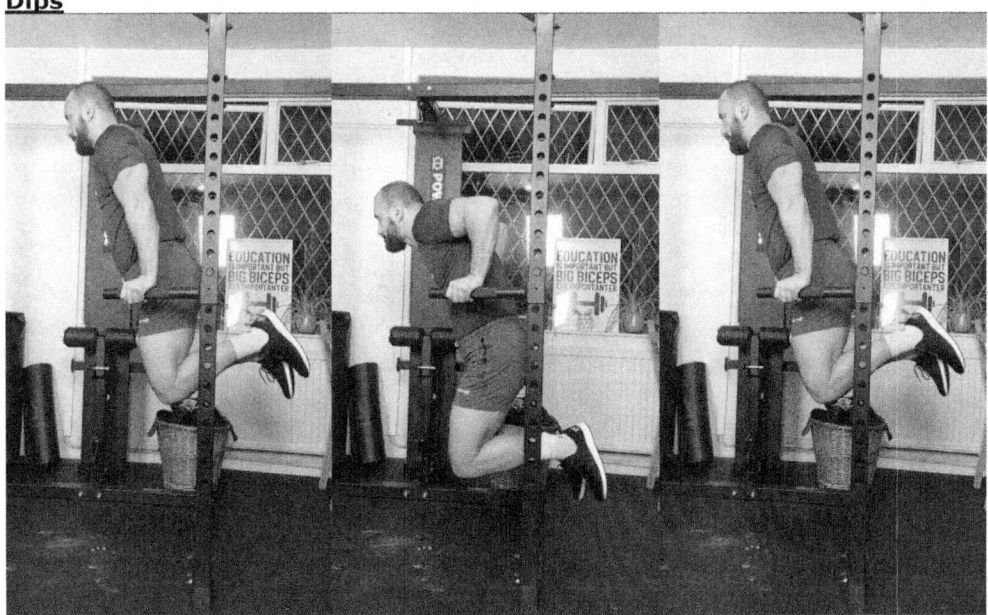

Dips

1. Grip the dipping bar with arms extended supporting your weight
2. Keeping your core engaged slowly lower yourself down until your upper arm is parallel to the floor
3. Extend your arms to return to the starting position in a controlled manner
4. Repeat for the desired number of repetitions

Stretching Guide

Flexibility is a fundamental component of fitness and the Commando90 programme promotes the use of stretching to assist with improving strength, fitness and health. There are different types of stretching with each type being deployed during certain times. The Commando90 Programme features **Dynamic Stretching** and **Passive Stretching**.

Dynamic Stretching
These are controlled repeated movements that put your muscles and joints through their range of motion. They should be part of a warm up routine. See the warm up video to see how dynamic stretches can be incorporated into the warm up.

Passive Stretching
These are stretches assisted by an external force and are typically held for 30 seconds. Passive stretching should be done after the work out.

This guide will display some recommended passive stretches.

Gently ease into position and once you feel the stretch hold for 30 seconds and breathe. Do not force the stretch to the point where it becomes painful!

Trapezius Stretch   Shoulder Stretch

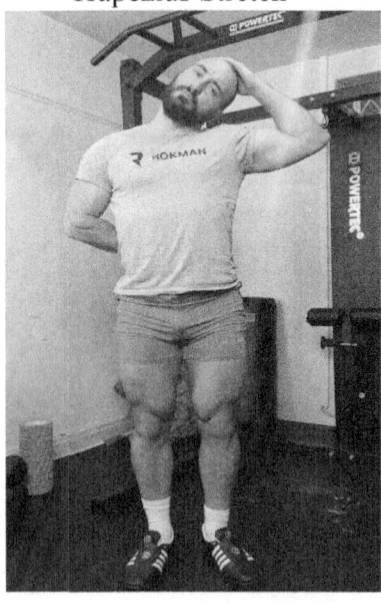

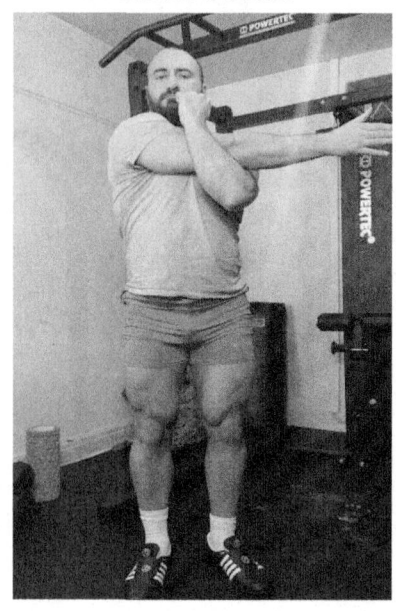

Chest Stretch

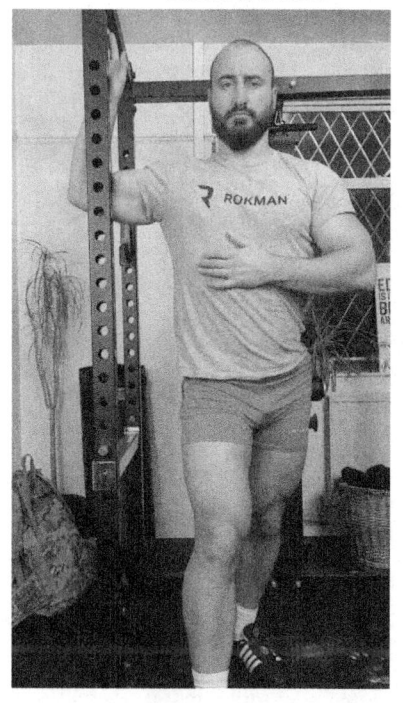

Back Stretches

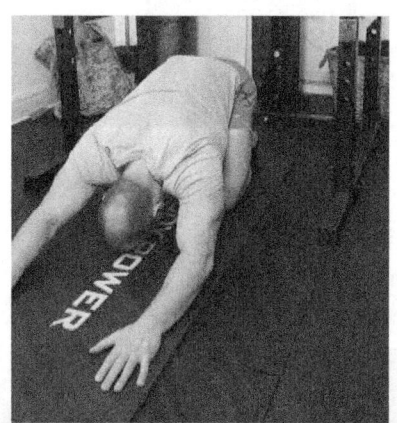

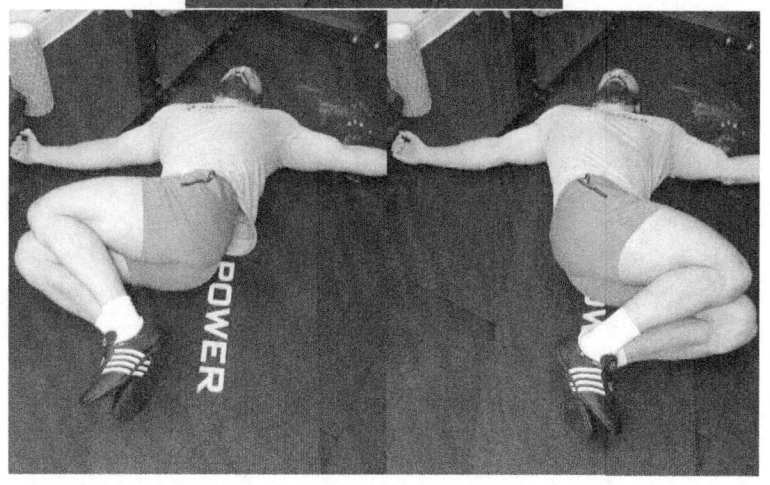

Hip Flexor Stretch

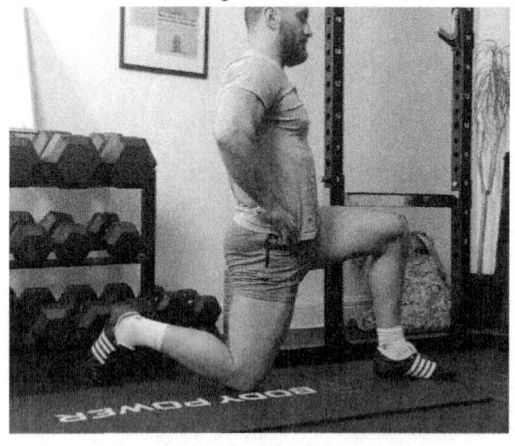

Quadricep Stretch

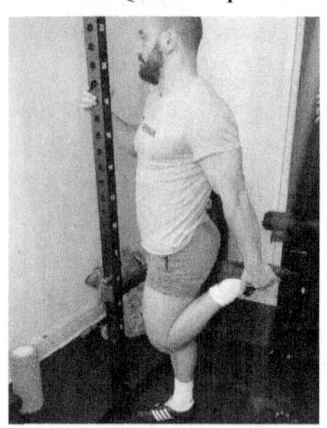

Hamstring & glute stretches

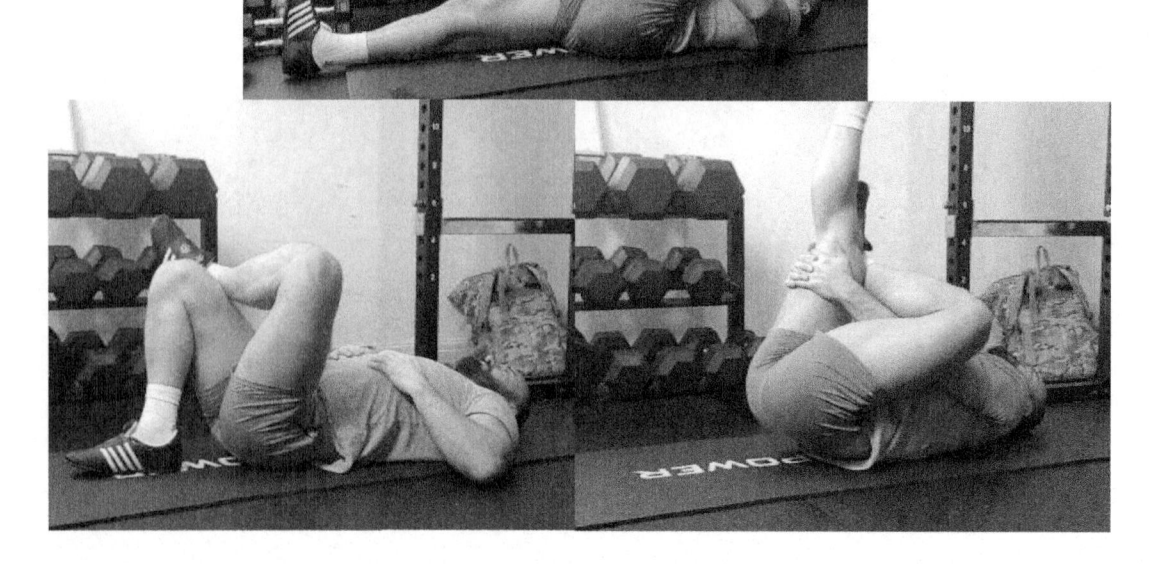

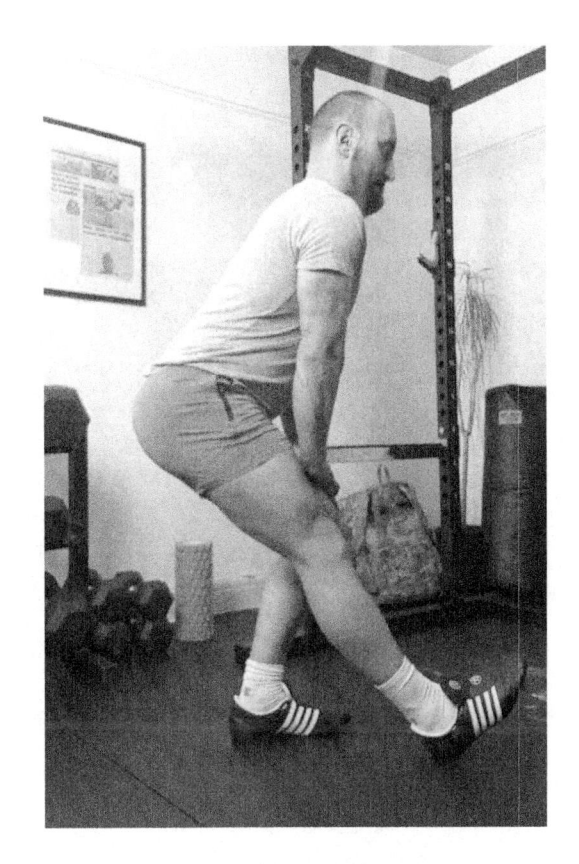

Calf Stretch

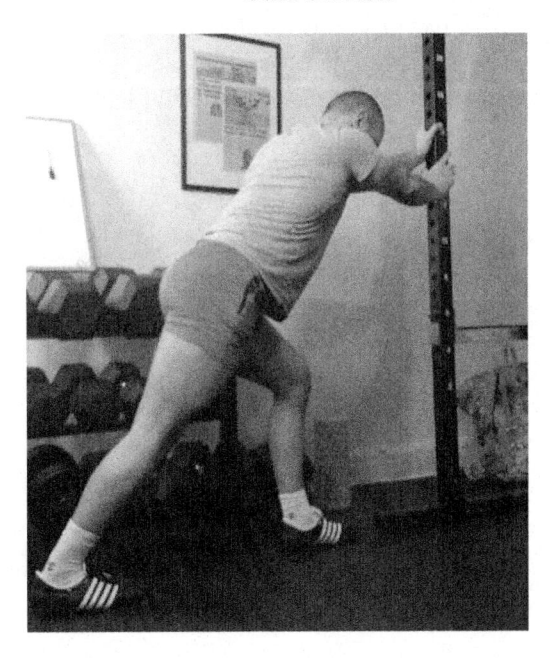

Author Profile

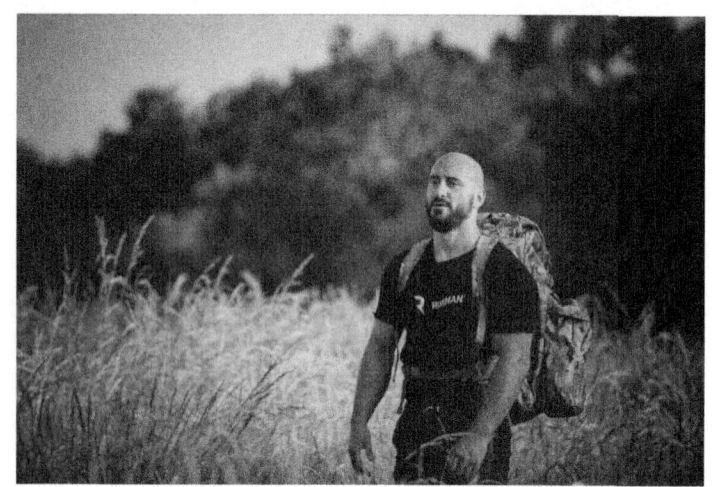

Image Credit:Rokman

Max Glover is a fitness enthusiast who now enjoys writing about his extreme challenges. The former Royal Marine has led a varied and unique life previously working as a maritime security operative and close protection officer and is now a proud ambassador of the mental resilience and running brand Rokman.

With stories to tell and training programmes to write - Max has pushed himself to the limits through a variety of disciplines - running, bodybuilding and calisthenics. Most recently raising thousands of pounds for charity by towing an 18-tonne truck for 2 miles (Furthest known distance), carrying a piano up a mountain, carrying 100kg for 100km (furthest known distance) and towing a 1.7 tonne car for 26.2 miles (smashing the world record at the time).

Max spends his down time relaxing with his family and cats and is most happy these days rucking with a heavy Bergen (military rucksack) enjoying the great outdoors... and is looking forward to sharing his next adventure with you!

More books from Max Glover:

Commando Runner

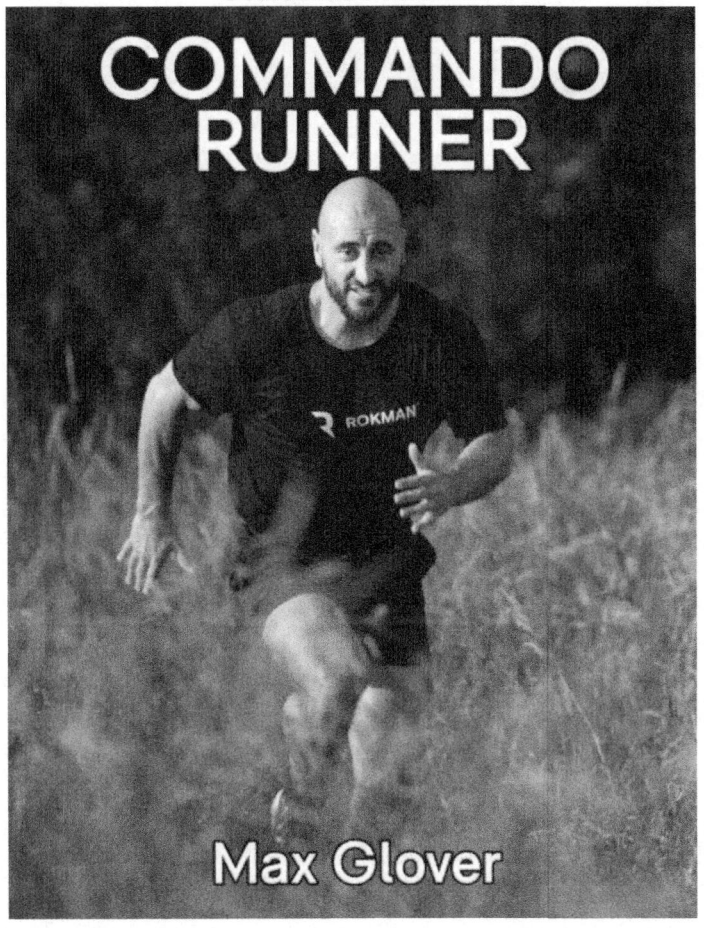

If you want to be the best, then start training like them. Use military training methods to improve your running and specifically your 1.5 mile run time.

Become The Elite

It's no secret - Royal Marines are renowned for their superior levels of physical fitness. This training programme uses methods employed by Commandos to achieve and maintain their elite performance. This guide will help If you are looking to join any branch of the military, run a 10k, obstacle course race, half marathon, if you are currently serving and looking to gain an edge over your peers or just improve your physical fitness.

- Comprehensive day by day training programme to follow - Be ready for anything
- How to optimise performance - Unlock the power of your mind
- Nutrition information - get the best out of your food
- Exercise and stretching guide - Activate and strengthen your muscles
- Fitness Testing - watch your times improve

Written by a former Royal Marine and extreme challenge athlete Max Glover

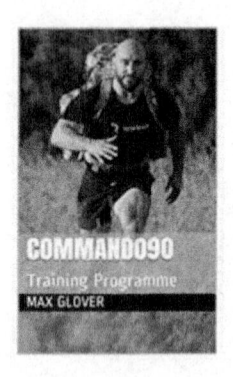

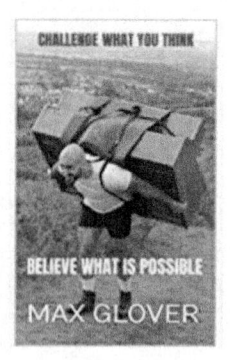

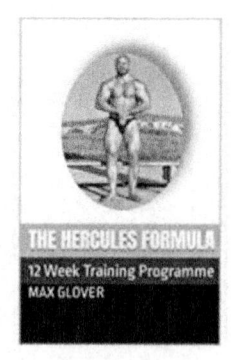

Commando90 – a 90 day no BS guide to obtain a Commando level of fitness. This is raw and basic, suitable for those who just want to follow a guide without any unnecessary distractions. Intense circuit training sessions for different abilities. Can be completed with bodyweight only and no fancy gym equipment.

Challenge What You Think, Believe What is Possible – Max Glover lets you into his mind while he completes unique challenges, such as carrying a piano up a mountain, towing a car for a marathon and much more. He explains how he trained for each challenge and also valuable lessons and insights from his time in the Royal Marines.

The Hercules Formula – This is a 12 week bodybuilding programme with the sole purpose of getting bigger and stronger using weights.

Image credits: Rokman www.rokman.co.uk @teamrokman

Instagram: @muscle.world.fitness

Printed in Great Britain
by Amazon